Nursing Care

at

Neonatology

The Complete Guide

ALEXANDRE CAREWELL

Table of contents

Introduction   17

- The magic of neonatology: 17
  understanding its importance

- The neonatal nurse: a central role   18

Chapter 1: The neonatal nurse's career   20
path

- How to prepare for a career in   20
  neonatology

- The key skills needed to excel in this   22
  field

- Career development: specialisations,   24
  teaching, management

Chapter 2: Diving into the world of   26
neonatology

- Origins and history of neonatology   26

- Structure and organisation of a   28
  neonatal unit

- Essential equipment: from incubators   30
  to cardiac monitors

Chapter 3: The day-to-day life of the   33
neonatal nurse

- The first few hours: admission and initial assessment   33

- Daily routine: care, feeding, monitoring   35

- Interaction with parents: a supportive and educational role   36

Chapter 4: Specific care for premature babies   38

- Understanding the physiology of the premature baby   38

- Common medical challenges: respiratory distress, jaundice, infections   39

- Appropriate care techniques: ventilation, phototherapy, nutrition   41

Chapter 5: Emergency situations and technical procedures   43

- Recognising an emergency situation in a neonatal unit   43

- Emergency procedures: neonatal CPR, intubation, venous lines   44

- Collaboration with the medical team: working in synergy   46

Chapter 6: Psychological and emotional dimensions   48

- Emotional resilience in the face of challenges   48

- Supporting parents: from compassion to education   50

- Stress management and the importance of self-care   51

Chapter 7: Teamwork   53

- The dynamics of the neonatology team   53
- Working with paediatricians, physiotherapists, psychologists and others   54
- Interprofessional communication: the key to cohesion   56

Chapter 8: Ethics and dilemmas in neonatology   58

- Introduction to medical ethics specific to neonatology   58
- Difficult decisions: when and how to intervene   59
- Working with families: respecting beliefs and wishes   61

Chapter 9: Research and innovation in neonatology   63

- The evolution of neonatal medicine: where do we stand?   63
- Taking part in research: the importance of staying at the cutting edge   65
- Technological innovations and their impact on care   66

Chapter 10: The role of the nurse in educating parents   69

- Preparing parents for discharge: education and training   69

- Handling difficult situations: bereavements, bad news, etc.   70

- Tools and resources for effective communication   72

Chapter 11: The importance of multidisciplinarity   75

- The role of each member of the neonatal medical team   75

- How to work effectively with different specialists   76

Chapter 12: Nutritional aspects in neonatology   79

- The importance of nutrition for newborn babies   79

- Different feeding methods: breastfeeding, enteral feeding, parenteral feeding, etc.   80

- Common nutritional challenges and solutions   82

Chapter 13: Pharmacology specific to neonatology   85

- Commonly used medicines and their indications   85

- Dosage, administration and monitoring of side effects   87

- Specific pharmacokinetics in neonates   88

Chapter 14: Complementary and alternative therapies   90

- Non-conventional approaches in neonatology: music therapy, therapeutic touch   90

- Studies and associated benefits   91

- How to integrate them safely   93

Chapter 15: The importance of family-centred care   95

- Involving parents in their child's care   95

- Holistic approach: considering the newborn in his or her family environment   97

Chapter 16: Neonatal safety   99

- Avoiding medical errors and guaranteeing patient safety   99

- The importance of reporting and safety culture   100

- Preventive measures and protocols in place   102

Chapter 17: Simulation and practical training   104

- The importance of simulation training in neonatology   104

- Common scenarios and how they prepare for clinical reality   105

- Feedback, debriefing and continuous improvement   107

Chapter 18: Leaving the neonatal unit and follow-up   110

- Preparing for discharge: assessing and educating parents   110

- The role of the nurse in post-neonatal monitoring   112

- The transition to paediatric care   113

Chapter 19: Neurodevelopment in neonatology   116

- Foundations of neurodevelopment in premature infants   116

- Impact of care and environment on the developing brain   118

- Strategies to support optimal neural development   120

Chapter 20: Palliative care in neonatology   122

- When and why they are needed   122

- How to approach end-of-life care with compassion   123

- Supporting families at this difficult time   125

Chapter 21: Environment and layout of the neonatal unit   127

- The importance of a suitable environment: light, sound, temperature   127

- Design and layout: from traditional units to centred family units   128

- Impact on the well-being of newborns, families and staff   130

Chapter 22: Infection management in neonatal units   132

- Prevention, detection and treatment of common infections   132

- Hygiene protocols   133

- Vaccination and prophylaxis in neonatology   135

Chapter 23: Atypical career paths: Gemini, malformations, etc.   137

- Managing complex and rare situations   137

- Care coordination for multiple situations   139

- Case studies and feedback   140

Chapter 24: Rehabilitation and physiotherapy in neonatology   143

- Importance of early mobilisation   143

- Techniques and routine operations   144

- Working with rehabilitation specialists   146

Chapter 25: Genetics and neonatology   148

- Introduction to genetics in neonatology   148

- Implications for diagnosis and care   149

- Genetic counselling and family support   151

Chapter 26: The importance of skin-to-skin contact and human contact   153

- The proven benefits of skin-to-skin contact   153

- Practical implementation and safety instructions   154

Chapter 27: Neonatal eye care   157

- Understanding retinopathy of prematurity   157

- Monitoring and treatment   158

- Prevention and awareness   159

Chapter 28: Cardiac care in neonatology   161

- Congenital heart defects: detection and management   161

- Working with paediatric cardiologists   162

- Case studies and research   164

Chapter 29: Neonatology and the environment   166

- Impact of pollutants and toxins on newborn babies   166

- Green initiatives in neonatal units   167

- Awareness-raising and education   169

Chapter 30: Dental care in neonatology   171

- The importance of oral health from birth   171

- Prevention and education for parents   172

- Working with paediatric dentists   174

Chapter 31: The challenges of pain and sedation   176

- Assessment and management of pain in newborns   176

- Judicious use of sedatives and analgesics   178

- Non-pharmacological techniques to relieve pain   179

Chapter 32: The role of music and art in neonatology   182

- Positive impact of music and art therapy   182

- Implementation in neonatal units   183

- Feedback and case studies   184

Chapter 33: The importance of continuity of care   187

- Ensuring a smooth transition between the different levels of care   187

- Collaboration between professionals for optimum continuity   189

- Implications for training and practice   190

Chapter 34: Continuing training and future prospects   193

- The importance of updating skills   193

- Advances in neonatology: being at the cutting edge of progress   194

- Career opportunities and specialisations   196

Conclusion   198

- The neonatal vocation: more than a job, a passion   198

- Encouraging the next generation: the future of neonatology   199

- The future of neonatology   201

- Technological advances on the horizon   202

- Current research and its implications for practice   204

- Vision of the future: where could neonatology take us in the coming decades?   205

« Neonatology: when humans arrive in mini version and you still have to install updates ! »

Introduction

The magic of neonatology: understanding its importance

From the very first moment that a newborn baby opens its eyes to the world, neonatology enters the scene. It's not just a branch of medicine or a series of medical protocols, it's the cradle where science meets art, where technique meets instinct, where every breath, every heartbeat is a miracle in itself.

Neonatology is the meeting of two worlds: the vast world of medicine and the tiny world of the newborn. And in this space, where gestures must be both precise and gentle, where decisions are made in the blink of an eye, a form of magic is hidden. This magic cannot be explained by figures, diagnoses or cutting-edge equipment alone. It lies in the ability to restore hope, to bring comfort, to create an unbreakable bond between a child and its parents, sometimes even before the latter have had a chance to hold it in their arms.

To truly understand the importance of neonatology, we need to recognise that it is much more than a medical discipline. It is the living expression of our collective desire to protect, care for and cherish life at its most fragile moments. Every neonatology professional, from the nurse who monitors the temperature of the incubator to the doctor who assesses vital signs, has a mission: to ensure that every newborn baby, whatever the challenges it faces, has the best possible chance of starting life.

If you take a closer look, the magic of neonatology is everywhere: in the warmth of a reassuring hand, in the gentle whisper of a lullaby sung in a baby's ear, in the pride of a team as they see a child leave the unit in full health. This magic is a reflection of our humanity, our dedication, and our deep understanding that every life, no matter how small, is of inestimable value.

The neonatal nurse :
a central role

At the heart of the neonatal unit, where life expresses itself with astonishing strength and fragility, the nurse is a pillar. Their presence is both reassuring and essential, because they are often the first human contact, the first gentle voice, the first touch for these babies who have just entered this world.

Much more than simple carers, neonatal nurses are watchers, guardians of life in the purest sense of the word. They are the silent witnesses to the first heartbeats, the first smiles, but also the moments of pain and challenge. They are the ones who, day after day, night after night, stand by these little creatures, offering them the care, attention and love they need.

Neonatal nurses do more than simply administer medication or monitor the baby's progress. He or she is a subtle interpreter of the signals that these newborns, still unable to speak, transmit. A slight variation in colour, a change in breathing rhythm, unusual behaviour - nothing escapes their expert eye. Thanks to their know-how and sensitivity, nurses are able to understand what babies are feeling and respond to their needs with remarkable precision.

But this central role goes far beyond purely medical care. Nurses also provide unfailing support to parents, who are often distraught and worried. It is the nurse who guides them, reassures them, informs them and accompanies them on this adventure full of emotions and uncertainties. Sometimes a confidant, sometimes an educator, the neonatal nurse forges deep and lasting ties with these families, becoming an essential link in the chain of care and love that surrounds these babies.

Being a neonatal nurse means embracing a life mission. It means choosing to be there, as life begins, to ensure that every baby, whatever their situation, gets the best possible start. It's choosing to put your heart, soul and skills at the service of these little lives, which in turn offer an inexhaustible source of inspiration, gratitude and wonder.

Chapter 1:
THE NURSE'S CAREER PATH IN NEONATOLOGY

How to prepare for a career in neonatology

Neonatology is a specialised and demanding field of medicine, but it also offers incomparable rewards. For those attracted to this field, preparing for a successful career in neonatology requires a combination of formal training, practical experience and personal development. Here are the steps you need to take to prepare yourself properly:

Initial training and specialisation :
Start by training in nursing or medicine, depending on whether you want to become a neonatal nurse or a neonatologist.
For doctors, once you've obtained your medical degree, you'll need to complete a residency in paediatrics, followed by a subspecialisation in neonatology.
Nurses should consider specialisation or certification in neonatal nursing.
Clinical experience :
Work in paediatric settings to learn about infant and child care.
Do placements or rotations in neonatal intensive care units (NICUs) to gain first-hand experience.
Developing soft skills :
Neonatology is not just about technical skills; it also requires compassion, patience and excellent communication skills. Training in

medical communication or emotional support can be beneficial.

Learn to work as part of a team. Neonatology is collaborative, often involving specialists, therapists, social workers and, of course, families.

Continuing education :

Medicine is changing fast. Attend regular conferences, workshops and courses to keep up to date with the latest research and techniques in neonatology.

Networking :

Join professional organisations related to neonatology. Not only will this keep you up to date with the latest trends, it will also give you the opportunity to meet mentors and colleagues with whom you can exchange ideas and experiences.

Taking care of yourself:

Neonatology can be emotionally demanding. It is essential to develop resilience strategies, whether through meditation, exercise, therapy or other methods to manage stress and avoid burn-out.

Participating in research :

If you're passionate about continuous improvement in neonatal care, consider getting involved in clinical studies or research projects. This can not only help advance the field, but also establish your reputation as an expert.

Ethics and cultural sensitivity :

Gain a solid understanding of the ethical issues involved in caring for newborn babies. In addition, given the diversity of the families you will meet, training in cultural sensitivity can also be invaluable.

Preparing for a career in neonatology takes time, effort and deep dedication. But for those who are called to this field, the privilege of accompanying newborns and their families during such crucial and emotional moments is a reward in itself.

Key skills
to excel in the field

Neonatology, like other medical specialties, requires a unique set of skills to ensure quality care for newborns and support for their families. To excel in this field, here are some essential skills to develop and refine:

- Clinical competence:
    - In-depth knowledge of neonatal physiology and pathology.
    - Ability to use and interpret sophisticated medical equipment.
    - Mastery of medical procedures specific to neonatology.
- Close observation:
    - Newborn babies cannot express their discomfort verbally. It is therefore crucial to have keen observation skills to detect subtle signs of distress or illness.
- Communication skills:
    - Explain complex medical situations clearly and calmly to parents and families.
    - Working effectively with a multidisciplinary team, including other doctors, nurses, therapists and social workers.
- Empathy and compassion:
    - Providing care with compassion, understanding and respecting the emotions of parents and families.

Stress management:

    Neonatology can be emotionally charged. Being able to manage stress and make quick decisions in emergency situations is essential.

Ethical competence:

    When faced with delicate situations such as end-of-life decisions or complex medical dilemmas, a solid understanding of ethical issues is crucial.

Continuing professional development:

    The willingness and ability to keep abreast of the latest research, techniques and practices in neonatology.

Organisational skills:

    Manage several patients efficiently, ensuring that each newborn receives the right care at the right time.

Cultural awareness:

    Understanding and respecting the different cultures and beliefs of families, as this can influence medical decisions and care preferences.

Emotional resilience:

    Be prepared to deal with emotionally intense situations, including the loss of patients or unexpected medical complications.

Patient-centred approach:

    Always prioritise the well-being of the newborn, ensuring that care is tailored to the individual needs of the patient and their family.

By combining these skills with a passion for the wellbeing of newborn babies and a commitment to clinical excellence, any neonatal professional will be well placed to provide exceptional care and make a significant difference to the lives of their patients and families.

Career development : specialisations, teaching, management

A career in neonatology, as in many medical fields, is rich and varied, allowing professionals to progress and specialise according to their interests and aspirations. Here are a few avenues for career development in this exciting field:

- More in-depth specialisations:
    - **Foetal medicine**: Focus on the diagnosis, consultation and treatment of foetal diseases.
    - **Neuroneonatology**: Specialisation in the neurological care of newborn babies, focusing on disorders of the brain and nervous system.
    - **Cardio-neonatology**: Focuses on congenital and acquired cardiac disorders in newborns.
- Clinical research :
    - Professionals can choose to become more involved in research, contributing to the advancement of knowledge, techniques and treatments in neonatology.
- Education and training :
    - Teaching the next generation of neonatologists or neonatal nurses in academic institutions.
    - Taking part in seminars, workshops and conferences as a speaker or trainer.
- Management and leadership :
    - **Head of Department**: Leading a team of neonatologists, nurses and other healthcare professionals in a neonatal intensive care unit.
    - **Hospital administrator**: Manages and supervises the operations of a neonatology department or specialist unit within a hospital or medical centre.

Health policy consultant: Working with policy-makers to influence and formulate policies relating to neonatal health.

Consultation :

As an expert in neonatology, providing consultancy services to other hospitals, clinics or institutions, guiding the development and improvement of clinical practice.

International development and humanitarian work :

Working with international organisations to improve neonatal care in developing or crisis regions.

Taking part in short-term medical missions to provide specialist care in needy regions.

Medical technology and innovation :

Working with the medical industry to develop and test new equipment, tools and technologies adapted to neonatal care.

Career development in neonatology offers many opportunities to specialise, take on leadership responsibilities, influence the future direction of the field and, above all, continue to make a significant difference to the lives of patients and their families.

Chapter 2:
DIVING INTO THE UNIVERSE NEONATOLOGY

Origins and history of neonatology

Neonatology, although considered a relatively recent medical speciality, has roots that stretch back over several centuries. The evolution of this speciality reflects the history of medicine itself, marked by technological advances, scientific discoveries and a growing commitment to the health of newborn babies.

Antiquity to the Renaissance:
Although caring for newborns has always been a human concern, methods were largely based on tradition, superstition and empirical observation. The writings of Hippocrates, Aristotle and other physicians of antiquity mention advice on the care of newborn babies.

17th and 18th centuries:
Incubators" made their appearance in Europe, inspired   by the incubators used in poultry farming. These first devices were rudimentary, but they showed a recognition of the vulnerability of premature babies.

19th century:
With the advent of the industrial era, exhibitions and fairs featured "incubators" with premature babies, drawing the public's attention to the needs of premature babies.

In 1880, Dr Étienne Stéphane Tarnier introduced the first hospital incubator for premature babies at the Maternité de Paris, marking a turning point in the medical care of newborn babies.

20th century:
> The first half of the century saw the advent of antibiotics, which considerably improved the survival rates of infected newborns.

> In the 1960s, with the advent of mechanical ventilation and continuous monitoring, neonatal intensive care units (NICUs) began to spread, offering specialist care to newborn babies.

> Over the decades, research and innovation have led to continuous improvements, particularly in the areas of neonatal nutrition, respiratory management and neuroprotection.

21st century:
> The emphasis is on a holistic approach to neonatal care. It's not just about survival, but also about the long-term quality of life of newborn babies.

> Evidence-based medicine is becoming the norm, with protocols and guidelines drawn up on the basis of rigorous clinical studies.

> The importance of family-centred care is recognised, with parents becoming more involved in care and decision-making.

Neonatology, as a dedicated medical speciality, is only a few decades old. However, the roots of concern and care for newborn babies go back to the dawn of time. The advances made over the centuries reflect not only developments in science and technology, but also a growing understanding and appreciation of the lives of the most vulnerable among us.

Structure and organisation
a neonatal unit

A neonatal unit is a specialised environment dedicated to the care of newborn babies, particularly those born prematurely, with congenital conditions or complications during or after birth. The structure and organisation of these units are designed to meet the unique needs of patients, while promoting efficiency, safety and collaboration between healthcare professionals.

Zoning :

Neonatal Intensive Care Unit (NICU): For newborns requiring intensive care, constant monitoring and specialist medical interventions.

Intermediate care unit: For newborns who no longer require intensive care, but who are not yet ready to be transferred to paediatrics or sent home.

Space for parents: Dedicated areas for parents to rest, feed and spend time with their baby.

Equipment and technology :

Incubators: Provide a controlled environment in terms of temperature, humidity and oxygen.

Ventilators: To assist the breathing of newborn babies.

Monitors: For continuous monitoring of heart rate, oxygen saturation, blood pressure and other vital parameters.

Phototherapy equipment: To treat neonatal jaundice.

Pumps and feeding equipment: To ensure nutrition for babies who cannot yet be breastfed or fed normally.

Staff :

Neonatologists: Paediatricians specialising in the care of newborn babies.

Neonatal nurses: Trained specifically to care for newborn babies, they play a central role in daily care and monitoring.

Respiratory therapists: Specialists in managing the respiratory needs of newborn babies.

Nutritionists: To ensure that every newborn baby receives appropriate nutrition.

Pharmacists: To manage and advise on medicines specific to neonatology.

Social workers and psychologists: to support families through the emotional and logistical challenges.

Specialist consultants: Including cardiologists, neurologists, paediatric surgeons, depending on patient needs.

Collaboration with other departments:

Close liaison with the maternity unit, paediatric surgery, laboratory, radiology and other departments to ensure comprehensive care.

Support for families :

Education programmes for parents on caring for newborn babies, breastfeeding, nutrition, etc.

Dedicated areas for breastfeeding, skin-to-skin contact and parental involvement in care.

Protocols and procedures :

Evidence-based guidelines for the management of a range of conditions and situations, from breathing and nutrition to infections.

The organisation of a neonatal unit reflects the complexity and specificity of newborn babies' needs. Every element - equipment, staff and procedures - is designed to ensure the best possible care for these particularly vulnerable patients and their families.

Essential equipment : from incubators to cardiac monitors

Neonatology is an area where technology and equipment play a crucial role. Each device is designed to meet the specific needs of newborn babies, particularly those who are premature or have health problems. This equipment not only saves lives but also improves the quality of life of babies during their stay in hospital.

Incubators :

Function: Incubators create a controlled environment for newborn babies, regulating temperature, humidity and, sometimes, oxygen. They also protect babies from infections, noise and excessive light.

Types: There are standard incubators, transportable incubators for transferring babies between hospitals, and incubators with integrated phototherapy systems.

Neonatal ventilators :

Function: These devices provide respiratory assistance for babies who cannot breathe independently. They are designed to deliver air and oxygen with a gentleness appropriate to the fragility of newborns' lungs.

Types : Positive pressure ventilators, CPAP (continuous positive airway pressure), high frequency ventilators.

Cardiac monitors :

Function: They continuously monitor the baby's heart rate, detecting any irregularities or arrhythmias.

Features: Equipped with screens to display heart rate in real time, alarms to signal anomalies, and sometimes integrated into global monitoring systems.

Oxygen saturation monitors :

Function: They measure the amount of oxygen in the baby's blood, often using a sensor placed on the foot or hand.

Features: These monitors use pulse oximetry technology and are essential for monitoring babies on ventilatory support.

Phototherapy equipment :

Function: Used to treat jaundice (hyperbilirubinemia) in newborn babies, they emit a blue light that transforms bilirubin into a form that the baby's body can eliminate.

Types : Phototherapy lamps, phototherapy mattresses, units integrated into incubators.

Feed pumps and probes :

Function: For babies who cannot be breastfed or who need specific nutrition, these devices enable milk or nutrient solutions to be administered directly into the stomach or intestine.

Types : Enteral feeding pumps, nasogastric tubes, orogastric tubes.

Heating tables :

Function: Unlike incubators, these open tables are heated to maintain the baby's body temperature. They are often used during medical procedures or for babies who need easy access for intensive care.

Precision, reliability and safety are at the heart of the design of this equipment. For neonatal healthcare professionals, mastery of these tools is essential to providing optimal care for newborn babies. Each device, whether simple or complex, has the potential to make a significant difference to the life of a baby and his or her family.

Chapter 3:
THE DAY-TO-DAY LIFE OF A NURSE IN NEONATOLOGY

The first few hours : admission and initial assessment

The admission of a newborn baby to a neonatal unit is a crucial period. The first few hours after birth are crucial to the child's health and well-being. The initial assessment plays an essential role in determining the baby's immediate needs and putting in place an appropriate care plan.

Arrival in the neonatal unit :

Transfer: Whether from the delivery room, another hospital unit or another establishment, the transfer must be carried out with care, often using a transportable incubator to ensure a stable environment for the newborn.

Welcome by the team: As soon as the baby arrives, the neonatology team is ready to intervene. This team generally includes a neonatologist, specialist nurses and, if necessary, a respiratory therapist.

Initial assessment :

Respiratory status: Assessment of breathing is essential. The frequency and rhythm of breathing are observed, as well as any cyanosis (bluish tinge to the skin) or other signs of respiratory distress.

Heart rate and tone: The regularity and strength of the pulse, as well as the baby's muscle tone, are assessed.

Body temperature: It is crucial to maintain a stable body temperature. Newborns are often placed under a heat source to prevent hypothermia.

Physical appearance: We look for any malformations, signs of prematurity or other anomalies.

Initial procedures :

Installation of monitors: The baby is often connected to heart and oxygen saturation monitors for continuous monitoring.

Blood samples: Blood samples can be taken to analyse blood sugar, bilirubin and other essential parameters.

Insertion of access ports: A peripheral venous line, umbilical catheter or feeding tube may be inserted as required.

Respiratory assistance: If necessary, the baby can be placed on a CPAP, ventilator or given supplementary oxygen.

Communication with the family :

Initial information: As soon as possible, parents are informed of their child's state of health, the interventions carried out and the short-term outlook.

Emotional support: admitting a newborn baby to the neonatal unit can be a traumatic experience for parents. Staff offer support, answer questions and provide reassurance wherever possible.

The first few hours in the neonatal unit are a medical ballet in which every step is vital. With skill and compassion, the neonatal team strives to ensure that every newborn receives the most appropriate care, laying the foundations for successful care in the days and weeks ahead.

The daily routine :
care, feeding, monitoring

As you enter the neonatal unit in the early hours of the morning, the soft murmur of the heart monitors and the subdued glow of the incubators create an atmosphere that is both soothing and intense. Here, every day is a delicate moment of care, feeding and constant monitoring, ensuring the well-being of the smallest and most vulnerable among us.

The morning often begins with a series of routine treatments. With gentle but confident movements, the nurse gently cleans each baby, changes nappies and gives gentle massages to stimulate circulation and well-being. These moments of physical contact are essential, as they promote not only the baby's physical health, but also the emotional bond, a crucial component of growth and development.

Feeding is central to this routine. Each newborn has specific nutritional needs. Some, who are ready to suckle, are breastfed directly by their mother or bottle-fed. For others, especially those born prematurely or with feeding difficulties, nutrition can be administered via a feeding tube. The nurses take the time to measure each quantity, ensuring that each baby receives exactly what he or she needs to grow and strengthen.

Monitoring is constant throughout the day. Every beep from a monitor, every little variation in the readings, is immediately noted and assessed. Heart monitors, oximeters and other equipment play a continuous melody, reflecting the vital rhythm of each baby. Doctors and nurses move from one incubator to the next, checking vital signs, adjusting medication or simply observing, always on the lookout for the slightest sign of distress or change.

But beyond the physical care, the daily routine in the neonatal unit is also made up of moments of tenderness. Parents, often anxious, find comfort in their child, gently caressing their tiny hand or whispering words of love in their ear. These moments, however brief, are essential to the emotional well-being of the baby and his family.

The day often ends as it began: calmly and resolutely. With every care, every meal and every watch, the neonatal team works tirelessly to ensure that every day is another step closer to home for these newborns. And on this journey, every routine, every daily gesture, is an act of love and dedication.

Interaction with parents : a support and education role

In the medicalised world of neonatology, where incubators buzz and monitors beep, one element remains essential and irreplaceable: the bond between parents and their newborn baby. For the nursing staff, facilitating and strengthening this bond is just as crucial a task as the medical care given to the babies. Interaction with parents has two dimensions: emotional support and education.

The birth of a child requiring neonatal care is often a shock for parents. The hospital setting, the tubes and wires, and the uncertainty about their baby's health can lead to fear, confusion and guilt. The neonatal nurse is often the first to establish a bond of trust with the parents, offering them an attentive ear and emotional support. She provides reassurance, guiding parents through their first contacts with their child, encouraging them to touch, talk and sing to their baby, reinforcing an essential bond.

But beyond support, the nurse also plays a crucial role in education. She introduces parents to the basic care of their newborn, teaches them to recognise signs of well-being or distress, and informs them about the various treatments and procedures their child may undergo. This transfer of knowledge is vital, as it enables parents to feel involved, competent and confident in their child's care, both in hospital and at home.

The education sessions can cover a variety of subjects, from nutrition to early stimulation and methods for calming a restless newborn. And while parents learn techniques and gestures, they also learn to read and understand their baby, to decipher every cry, every smile, every movement.

There are also times when the nurse needs to address more sensitive issues, such as medical complications, long-term perspectives or difficult treatment decisions. At these times, honesty, compassion and clarity are essential.

Interactions with parents in neonatology are a delicate dance between the head and the heart. The nurse brings knowledge and skills, but also empathy and compassion. And through this prism, she sees not only a baby in need of medical care, but also a family in the making, trying to find its way in a new and unfamiliar world. By supporting and educating, she becomes a beacon for these families, guiding them through the storms and into calmer waters.

Chapter 4:
SPECIFIC TREATMENTS
PREMATURE BABIES

Understanding the physiology
of the premature baby

Discovering the world before term makes each premature baby a unique being, with a physiology that is particularly adapted to his or her condition. Understanding this physiology opens a window onto a world where every bodily function is at the crossroads of adaptation and vulnerability.

Depending on their gestational age, premature babies have not had time to perfect all the physiological mechanisms essential to life outside the womb. Their thin, translucent skin, for example, is less effective at retaining heat, making them more susceptible to hypothermia. To compensate, the premature baby may have a higher heart rate and metabolic rate, in an attempt to produce more heat.

Its respiratory system, often the most affected by prematurity, is characterised by less developed lungs and a deficit in surfactant, the substance that prevents the alveoli from collapsing. This makes breathing more difficult for premature babies and exposes them to pathologies such as hyaline membrane disease.

The digestive system of the premature baby is also immature. Their stomachs are small and their ability to digest and absorb nutrients is limited. What's more, the coordination between sucking, swallowing and breathing is not always perfected, which can make feeding by breast or bottle initially difficult.

The immune system is another area of vulnerability. Premature babies, who have not benefited from the total intake of maternal antibodies that occurs at the end of pregnancy, are more susceptible to infections. Fortunately, colostrum, rich in protective agents, provides an initial defence barrier when the mother is able to breastfeed.

From a neurological point of view, the premature baby's brain is still developing. Cerebral structures, such as the ventricles and white matter, are particularly sensitive to attack, whether mechanical, such as haemorrhage, or biochemical, such as anoxia.

Despite these physiological challenges, premature babies also have an incredible capacity for resilience and adaptation. With the right care and a suitable environment, the majority of these babies catch up with their full-term peers, both physically and neurologically.

As we delve into the physiology of the premature baby, we discover a world where fragility rubs shoulders with strength, where every day is a victory and every step forward a celebration. It's a poignant reminder of the wonder of life and the incredible capacity of the human body to adapt and overcome obstacles.

Common medical challenges : respiratory distress, jaundice, infections

The neonatal unit is often compared to a zone of high vigilance where, at every second, medical teams face demanding medical challenges that are crucial to the lives of newborn babies. Three in particular stand out: respiratory distress, jaundice and infections.

1. Respiratory distress :

The first major test for many premature babies is the very act of breathing. The immature lungs may lack surfactant, the precious compound that keeps the alveoli open. This deficiency can lead to hyaline membrane disease, where the lungs cannot expand properly. Affected babies often show rapid breathing, bluish skin and retractions. To cope, exogenous administration of surfactant and support by mechanical ventilation may be necessary.

2. Jaundice :

Almost trivial in its frequency, but not without risks, jaundice is due to the accumulation of bilirubin in the blood. Bilirubin, produced when red blood cells break down, is normally eliminated by the liver. But in newborn babies, especially premature ones, this elimination can be slowed down. The skin and eyes then take on a yellowish tinge. In most cases, phototherapy, in which the baby is placed under a special light, is enough to solve the problem. However, if ignored or poorly treated, severe jaundice can lead to irreversible brain damage.

3. Infections :

The immune system of newborn babies, particularly premature babies, is still developing, making them more vulnerable to bacterial, viral or fungal infections. These infections can be acquired in utero, during delivery or after birth. The symptoms are often subtle: lethargy, poor food intake or thermal instability. The consequences, however, can be serious, requiring rapid intervention with antibiotics or other drugs. Prevention, through strict hygiene and sometimes prophylactic administration of antibiotics, is essential.

Faced with these challenges, the role of neonatal medical teams is not only to diagnose and treat accurately, but also to anticipate, educate and support families. Because every medical challenge is also an emotional journey for parents, and guiding them through this rollercoaster is an integral part of comprehensive newborn care.

Appropriate care techniques: ventilation, phototherapy, nutrition

In the neonatal arena, where the smallest patients fight for their lives, care techniques specifically adapted to their needs are the shield and sword of the medical teams. Ventilation, phototherapy and feeding are the three pillars of these techniques, each responding to specific medical challenges.

1. Ventilation :
The ability to breathe is vital, yet it is one of the main difficulties faced by premature babies. Their immature respiratory system often requires assistance:

Non-invasive ventilation: Methods such as CPAP (Continuous Positive Airway Pressure) keep the airways open by providing constant air pressure, making it easier to breathe without the need for intubation.

Mechanical ventilation: For more severe cases, a machine takes over the baby's breathing through a tracheal intubation. The key is to carefully adjust the pressure, volume and frequency to minimise lung damage.

Surfactant : This substance, administered directly into the lungs, helps prevent alveolar collapse, which is common in babies with hyaline membrane disease.

2. Phototherapy :
Faced with the silent threat of jaundice, phototherapy is a gentle but effective technique:

Blue light: Babies are placed under a special blue light. This light transforms bilirubin, which accumulates in the blood and skin, into a more soluble form that can be eliminated through urine and faeces.

41

Fibre optics: In some cases, a fibre-optic blanket or light mattress is used, offering the advantage of less interrupted contact between parents and child.

3. Power supply :

Nutrition is the fuel of development. For a premature baby, nutrition is not just a necessity, it's a therapy:

Enteral feeding: Starting with small quantities, breast milk or a special formula is administered directly into the baby's stomach or intestine using a feeding tube.

Breastfeeding and bottle-feeding: Encouraged as soon as the baby is ready, these actions strengthen the parent-child bond and encourage better coordination of sucking and swallowing.

Supplementation: Premature babies may need extra nutrients to support their rapid growth, added either to breast milk or to formula.

Using these techniques, the neonatal team works tirelessly to meet the specific needs of newborn babies. Each intervention is a combination of art and science, guided by an in-depth knowledge of the physiology of the premature baby and an unshakeable determination to give each child the best possible start in life.

Chapter 5:
EMERGENCY SITUATIONS
AND TECHNICAL GESTURES

Recognising an emergency situation in neonatology

In neonatology, emergency situations can evolve rapidly, transforming a stable situation into a life-threatening crisis in the blink of an eye. The ability to recognise and respond quickly to these emergencies is essential to ensure the safety and well-being of fragile newborns. Here are some warning signs and symptoms that indicate an emergency situation:

1. Respiratory distress :
   - Rapid or shallow breathing, often accompanied by a grinding sound.
   - Retractions, where the skin between the ribs, around the neck or under the ribs is pulled with each breath.
   - Cyanosis, a bluish tinge to the skin, particularly around the lips and fingers, indicating low oxygenation.
   - Apnoeas, pauses in breathing lasting more than 20 seconds.
2. Cardiovascular instability :
   - Bradycardia, a significant drop in heart rate.
   - Palpitations or cardiac arrhythmias.
   - Low perfusion, indicated by cold, pale or mottled skin and prolonged capillary refill times.
3. Neurological problems :
   - Convulsions, which may manifest as jerky movements, eye rotation or rigidity.
   - Lethargy or a lack of responsiveness, where the baby is less responsive to stimuli.

Extreme irritability or inconsolable crying.
4. Diet and gastrointestinal problems :
Repeated refusal to feed or frequent regurgitation.
Abdominal distension or hardness.
Bilious, greenish-coloured vomiting, indicating possible intestinal obstruction.
Blood in the stools.
5. Signs of infection :
Unstable body temperature, either fever or hypothermia.
Lethargy or irritability.
Low food intake.
Pale or greyish complexion.

Rapid intervention is key in neonatology. Early recognition of emergency signs, followed by immediate medical intervention, can make the difference between a favourable outcome and serious complications. That's why the ongoing education and training of carers, and the establishment of clear emergency protocols, are essential in this delicate and crucial area of medicine.

Emergency procedures: neonatal CPR, intubation, venous lines

Neonatology, with its fragile patients and their specific needs, demands rapid, expert intervention in emergencies. Neonatal emergency procedures require specialised training and a perfect command of techniques, because every second counts.

1. Neonatal CPR (cardiopulmonary resuscitation) :
When a newborn is not breathing or has no perceptible pulse at birth, neonatal CPR is performed.
Initial assessment: Rapid examination of the baby's breathing, muscle tone and colour.

Ventilation: If the baby is not breathing or is breathing irregularly, ventilation is the priority. Use a face mask and bag to administer insufflations.

Chest compressions: If the pulse remains below 60 beats per minute despite effective ventilation, start chest compressions, combined with ventilation at a ratio of 3:1.

Medication: If the above measures are not effective, drugs such as epinephrine may be administered.

2. Intubation :

When ventilation with a mask and bag is not sufficient, or when prolonged ventilation is required, intubation may be necessary.

Probe selection: Choose the appropriate probe size for the newborn.

Positioning: Place the baby in the "rose scent" position with a slight extension of the neck.

Insertion: Insert the endotracheal tube into the trachea and confirm its position by auscultation and detection of exhaled CO_2.

Securing: Secure the probe to prevent accidental movement.

3. Venous routes :

To administer medicines, nutrients or fluids, it is sometimes necessary to establish venous access in newborns.

Umbilical vein: One of the most common methods used in newborns is the use of umbilical veins. Umbilical vein catheters can provide rapid access for the administration of drugs and fluids.

Peripheral vein: For short-term access, a peripheral vein, usually in the arm or leg, can be used.

PICC (Peripherally Inserted Central Catheter): For longer access or to administer drugs that cannot be administered via a peripheral route, a PICC can be placed.

Every neonatal procedure requires precision, expertise and attention to detail. In these moments of urgency, the medical team must not only possess technical skills, but must also work together in synchrony, always ensuring the well-being and safety of the newborn.

Collaboration with the medical team: working in synergy

In the intense and often unpredictable world of neonatology, interprofessional collaboration is more than just a concept: it's a vital necessity. The multidisciplinary nature of neonatal care requires synergy between various health professionals to ensure the best possible outcome for these little patients.

1. Understanding roles :
Each member of the team has a distinct and essential role.
- **Neonatologist: A** medical specialist who oversees all care and makes critical decisions about the care of newborn babies.
- **The neonatal nurse:** Provides direct care to the newborn, constantly monitors his or her condition and communicates his or her observations to the team.
- **Respiratory therapists:** Experts in ventilation and respiratory support, they play an essential role when babies have lung problems.
- **The pharmacist:** Ensures that medicines are appropriate for the patient, in the right doses and without dangerous interactions.

2. Effective communication :
In this high-voltage environment, clear and rapid communication is vital. Teams need to regularly review

patients' conditions, discuss treatment plans and ensure that everyone is on the same wavelength.

3. Collegial decisions :
Neonatal situations are often not black and white. This requires the team to come together to discuss the best management strategies, weighing up the benefits and risks of each decision.

4. Joint training and simulations :
Organising joint training sessions, where different healthcare professionals learn and train together, reinforces mutual understanding of roles and improves coordination in real-life situations.

5. Emotional support :
Faced with situations that are often emotionally charged, it is crucial that team members support each other, recognising the value and importance of each other's work.

6. Inclusion of parents :
The medical team must also work closely with the parents, regarding them as essential partners in their child's care. Their involvement and education about neonatal care are crucial.

Neonatology is an area where the life of a newborn baby can depend on the fluidity with which the medical team works together. It is this alchemy, this synergy between professionals, that transforms a group of individuals into a cohesive unit, capable of overcoming challenges and providing the best possible care to these vulnerable patients.

Chapter 6:
PSYCHOLOGICAL DIMENSIONS AND EMOTIONAL

Emotional resilience in the face of challenges

The neonatal unit is a world of marked contrasts: moments of pure joy when a baby passes a medical milestone, and moments of profound sadness when unexpected complications arise. It's a place where victories are celebrated with passion and losses mourned with equal intensity. For the healthcare professionals who work there, developing emotional resilience is not only desirable, but essential.

1. Understanding the nature of the work :
Neonatal care, by its very nature, involves working with some of the most vulnerable patients. Nurses and doctors must be prepared to deal with situations where, despite their best efforts, the outcome can be unpredictable.

2. The practice of self-care :
It is essential that healthcare professionals take time for themselves, whether through hobbies, exercise, meditation or any other activity that helps them recharge their batteries.

3. Finding support :
Sharing experiences and feelings with colleagues or through support groups can help deal with difficult emotions. They understand the specific challenges of the job and can offer a valuable perspective.

4. Clinical supervision :
Having regular sessions with a trained professional, to discuss difficult cases and the emotional impact they can have, is a beneficial strategy for many.

5. Continuing education :
Education and training can reinforce a sense of competence, reducing anxiety and uncertainty in tense situations.

6. Accepting your emotions :
It's normal to feel a range of emotions, from moments of ecstasy to moments of deep grief. Recognising and accepting these emotions, rather than repressing them, is an essential step in developing resilience.

7. Setting limits :
Knowing when to say "no" or when to take a day off is crucial to avoiding burnout.

8. Remember why :
Regularly returning to the fundamental reason for choosing this profession can help to put the challenges into perspective. The joy of helping a newborn thrive is immeasurable.

Neonatal professionals have incredible strength, combined with great sensitivity. This unique combination enables them to provide exceptional care. But it can also make them particularly vulnerable to emotional trauma. By actively cultivating resilience, they can continue to offer their valuable support while looking after their own emotional well-being.

Supporting parents :
from compassion to education

Entering the world of neonatology is often an unexpected journey for many parents. Dreams of gentle lullabies and first smiles are suddenly interspersed with the beeping of monitors, the bluish glow of phototherapy and the constant hum of incubators. For parents, this new world is overwhelming, complex and frightening. And this is where the neonatal nurse plays a pivotal role, providing not only medical skills but also indispensable human support.

It all starts with compassion. Parents often find themselves overwhelmed by a tide of conflicting emotions: hope, fear, guilt, love. Recognising their vulnerabilities, listening to them without judgement and offering them a space to express their feelings is essential. A simple gesture, like a hand on the shoulder, can offer immeasurable comfort.

But support does not stop at compassion. Education also plays a crucial role. Parents are eager to understand what's going on, to decode complex medical terms, to learn about the machines that surround their child and to interpret the signals their baby sends them. As intermediaries between the medical world and the world of parents, nurses are ideally placed to bridge this gap. By explaining clearly, demonstrating procedures and, above all, encouraging parents to ask questions, they gradually transform them from anxious bystanders into active partners in care.

Support for parents is also rooted in respect for their role. Despite the medical environment, it is vital to remind them that these are their children. This means encouraging them to participate in daily care, to establish a skin-to-skin bond, to sing for their baby, and to celebrate every little victory.

And finally, it is essential to support these parents as they prepare to leave the hospital. Leaving the neonatal unit is a major step, full of anticipation, but also apprehension. Equipping them with the knowledge and confidence to care for their child at home strengthens their ability to fully embrace their parental role.

Supporting parents in neonatology is a delicate dance between compassion and education. It's a shared journey, where every step, every smile, every tear forges an alliance with the ultimate goal of seeing each baby flourish. And on this journey, the nurse is guide, teacher and companion all rolled into one.

Stress management and the importance of self-care

Working in neonatology is not a task for the faint-hearted. Every day, nurses are confronted with delicate situations where the stakes are high and emotions run high. In this tumultuous environment, stress management and self-care are not just luxuries; they become a vital necessity, both for the personal well-being of the nurse and for the quality of care provided to the little patients and their families.

Stress, although often perceived as an enemy, is in fact the body's natural response to challenges. It sharpens the senses, prepares us for action and can even improve performance in the short term. However, when it becomes chronic, it can erode mental, physical and emotional health, leading to burnout, depression and other illnesses.

Self-care means recognising and responding to your own needs. It's a proactive way of keeping your emotional reservoir full so you can give to others without burning out.

Here's how nurses can incorporate this essential practice into their routine:

1. Self-awareness: It's essential to listen to yourself, recognise the signs of stress or fatigue and act accordingly. Taking a moment to breathe, meditate or simply stretch can sometimes make all the difference.

2. Healthy limits: Understand that saying "no" or asking for help is not a sign of weakness, but rather an affirmation of your own limits.

3. Diet and exercise: Eating well and exercising regularly are not only good for the body, but also for the mind. They can help manage stress and improve mood.

4. Pause and disconnect: In an always-connected world, it's crucial to allow yourself moments of disconnection, whether by taking a holiday or simply going for a walk without your phone.

5. Social support: Sharing your experiences and feelings with colleagues, friends or family can provide invaluable perspective and reassurance.

6. Ongoing training: Sometimes stress comes from feeling like you're not up to the job. Continuing training can boost your self-confidence and broaden your skills.

7. Passions and hobbies: Having an activity outside work that brings joy can serve as an escape and recharge the batteries.

8. Professional advice: When stress or emotions become too much to bear, it may be useful to consult a mental health professional.

In neonatology, where every moment counts, taking care of yourself is not a selfish act, but a duty. It is by recharging their batteries that nurses can offer the best of themselves, navigating with grace and efficiency through the storms and serene moments of this unique profession.

Chapter 7:
WORKING IN A TEAM

Team dynamics
in neonatology

In neonatology, where the beeping of machines merges with the soft whispers of parents and the cries of infants, one constant remains: the dynamic of the team. Like a well-orchestrated symphony, each member plays a unique but essential note, contributing to a melody that is greater than the sum of its parts.

The neonatal team is a kaleidoscope of skills, cultures and perspectives. From nurses to neonatologists, nutritionists, physiotherapists, social workers and technicians, each professional contributes their expertise to ensure the most comprehensive care for premature or sick babies.

This diversity, while an asset, is also a challenge. Each member must not only excel in their own field, but also understand and appreciate the role of others. Communication then becomes the cornerstone of this dynamic. Exchanges need to be clear, concise and respectful, turning potential differences into opportunities for mutual learning.

Trust is another key element. In an environment where decisions often have to be taken quickly, each member must have confidence in the ability of others to act competently and ethically. This trust is forged over time, through successes, trials and challenges overcome together.

But beyond skills and communication, there's heart. The neonatal team is united by a common passion: the well-being of the smallest and most vulnerable babies. This deep commitment creates an unbreakable bond between its members. It's not unusual to see teams supporting each other through difficult times, celebrating small victories together, or sharing a moment of contemplation when sadness strikes.

Finally, the team dynamic is also fuelled by a constant desire to improve. Ongoing training, case discussions and practice reviews are moments when the team comes together to reflect, learn and innovate.

The cohesion and complementarity of the neonatal team is the beating heart of the unit. It is living proof that, even in the most critical moments, collaboration, respect and passion can work miracles.

Working with paediatricians, physiotherapists, psychologists and others

Neonatology is a complex world, where every day brings challenges, but also hopes and successes. To navigate this sea of uncertainty, inter-professional collaboration is not only recommended, it's vital. Each professional brings his or her own specific expertise to bear in creating a holistic approach to the care of newborn babies and their families.

Paediatricians are often on the front line, contributing their in-depth knowledge of neonatal physiology and diseases. They guide the team through medical protocols, diagnoses and treatment plans. Their experience is essential for assessing the infant's health, anticipating potential complications and adapting care accordingly.

Physiotherapists, or kinesiologists, play a key role in the care of infants with specific respiratory needs or motor challenges. Their expertise helps to improve lung function, promote better oxygenation and stimulate early motor development, essential for a good start in life.

Psychologists have a special role to play. They support not only the emotional well-being of parents, who are often overwhelmed by anxiety, guilt or grief, but also that of the medical team. They offer a place to listen, help detect signs of psychological distress and suggest strategies for managing emotions and stress.

The collaboration doesn't stop there. **Dieticians** ensure that each infant receives nutrition tailored to his or her specific needs. **Social workers** help families navigate social or financial challenges, and access necessary resources. **Pharmacists** ensure that medicines are administered safely and effectively.

This collaboration is rooted in communication. Team meetings, case discussions and handovers are all good opportunities to exchange information, ask questions and make informed decisions. It's a delicate dance, where everyone has to listen, respect each other's expertise and constantly seek to learn.

Ultimately, this inter-professional collaboration has just one aim: to give newborn babies the best possible chance of survival and development. Because in the world of neonatology, every skill, every gesture counts, and it's together, by pooling our strengths and knowledge, that we can achieve the greatest miracles.

Interprofessional communication: the key to cohesion

At the heart of a department as delicate as neonatology, where every second counts and every decision can have irreversible consequences, lies an essential element: inter-professional communication. It is this communication that weaves the fabric on which the harmonious care of babies and their families depends.

Communication between healthcare professionals is not simply an exchange of information. It is a nuanced dialogue that requires clarity, precision, active listening and mutual respect. Each member of the team, whether nurse, paediatrician, physiotherapist, psychologist or other, holds a piece of the jigsaw, and it is only by putting these pieces together that we can obtain a complete and clear picture of the situation.

The value of this communication can be seen in a number of ways. Firstly, it ensures continuity of care. When one professional accurately conveys information about a newborn baby's state of health, the next team member can take over without losing time. This fluidity is crucial, particularly at critical moments.

Secondly, it facilitates collaborative decision-making. Faced with complex situations where several approaches are possible, the team needs to work together to choose the best course of action. These multidisciplinary discussions make it possible to combine expertise, assess the benefits and risks of each option, and reach an informed consensus.

But interprofessional communication goes beyond the purely clinical aspects. It also plays a vital role in maintaining team cohesion. Working in an environment as demanding as neonatology can generate tensions. Open communication helps to defuse potential conflicts, clarify misunderstandings and strengthen the bonds between team members.

It also creates a space for professional growth. By exchanging experiences, asking questions and sharing knowledge, professionals enrich each other. These interactions, far from being mere conversations, become opportunities for learning, questioning and innovation.

Interprofessional communication is the lifeblood of the neonatal unit. It reflects a fundamental reality: in this world where the lives of the smallest and most fragile babies are at stake, it's only by working together, speaking the same language and sharing the same values, that we can offer the best possible care.

Chapter 8:
ETHICS AND DILEMMAS
IN NEONATOLOGY

Introduction to medical ethics specific to neonatology

Medical ethics, the moral compass that guides caregivers in their choices and actions, takes on a particularly poignant dimension in neonatology. In this speciality, where life often begins with a struggle, every decision is fraught with consequences and is marked by intrinsic ethical dilemmas.

Neonatology is the scene of situations where the line between life and death can be infinitely tenuous. When faced with a premature newborn or one suffering from a serious pathology, at what point do we intervene, and up to what point? The delicate balance between preserving life at all costs and not imposing unnecessary suffering or a diminished quality of life is at the heart of ethical concerns. Several fundamental questions arise:

Therapeutic overkill: How far should we go in caring for a newborn baby? Is there a point at which we have to recognise that continuing invasive treatments may be more harmful than beneficial?

Parental autonomy: While it is essential to respect parents' wishes and beliefs, how can their autonomy be reconciled with what is medically appropriate for the child? And what should be done when parents' beliefs conflict with medical recommendations?

Quality of life: How is a newborn's future quality of life assessed and taken into account when making medical decisions? Is it ethical to make decisions

58

based on predictions, often uncertain, about the future challenges the child may face?

Limited resources: In a world where medical resources are often limited, how is the allocation of neonatal intensive care decided? What criteria should be used to determine who receives care in situations of scarcity?

Neonatology, by its very nature, regularly confronts carers with these dilemmas. Every decision is tinged with a profound sense of humanity, a constant questioning of what is "right" or "good". This is a field where ethics is not an abstract reflection, but a daily reality, embodied in the eyes of a newborn baby, in the hope of a parent, in the hand that administers care.

Ethics in neonatology is therefore an invitation to deep reflection, humility and informed decision-making, always in the interests of the newborn and his or her family. It is a reminder that behind every medical act there is a story, a life, and an immense responsibility.

Difficult decisions : when and how to intervene

Neonatology is a world where every decision can carry a lot of weight. Between medical science, the wishes of the parents and the well-being of the newborn, healthcare professionals are often navigating murky waters, trying to find the best course to follow. When a baby's medical situation is complex or uncertain, making the 'right' decision can be a major challenge.

Medical assessment: It all starts with a thorough medical assessment. What is the newborn's current situation? What are its immediate needs? How will it develop in the short and long term? Although medicine can provide many answers, it is also fraught with uncertainty. It is crucial that carers recognise and communicate these uncertainties to the team and to the parents.

Consideration of parents: Parents are their child's main advocates. Their wishes, hopes, fears and convictions must be listened to and taken into account. This active listening forms the basis of a relationship of mutual trust, which is essential for joint decision-making.

Ethical dilemmas: In some cases, the path to take is not clearly defined. Continuing aggressive treatment may prolong life, but at what cost to the baby? Sometimes the most compassionate choice is to provide palliative care, focusing on comfort rather than cure. These decisions, which are profoundly ethical, require reflection, dialogue and often the support of an ethics committee.

Transparent communication: When difficult decisions are on the horizon, communication between all those involved is vital. Doctors, nurses and other health professionals need to share information in a clear, transparent and empathetic way, enabling parents to understand the situation and take an active part in it.

Psychological support: Neonatal decisions can have a profound emotional impact, not only on parents but also on carers. Psychological support, whether from psychologists, social workers or support groups, is essential to help everyone navigate these tumultuous waters.

Acknowledging bereavement: In situations where the death of a newborn is imminent or has already occurred, acknowledging and honouring the bereavement process is crucial. Each member of the team must approach this stage with sensitivity, offering parents the space, time and support they need to cope with their loss.

Decision-making in neonatology is a delicate art, a balance between science, ethics and humanity. In this constant quest for the best for the newborn and his or her family, every professional is called upon to demonstrate competence, compassion and courage.

Working with families : respecting beliefs and wishes

The neonatal unit, with its subdued lighting, soft intermittent beeps and fragile occupants, is a place of strong emotions. For families, it's a place where hope and anxiety coexist. In this context, collaboration between carers and families becomes a central pillar of care. At the heart of this alliance is the need to recognise and respect parents' beliefs and wishes.

Active listening: First and foremost, it's important to listen. Parents, often overwhelmed by the situation, need to feel that their fears, hopes and convictions are being heard. Listening is more than just listening: it involves being fully present, being open-minded and responding with empathy.

Open dialogue: Once you've listened, dialogue can begin. This involves an honest exchange where medical information is shared clearly, allowing parents to understand their child's situation. In return, healthcare professionals have the opportunity to hear and understand the parents' perspectives and wishes.

Taking beliefs into account: Each family comes with its own cultural, religious and ethical baggage. Whether it's a belief in the value of life, a ritual practice or an alternative approach to care, these beliefs must be recognised and, as far as possible, incorporated into the care plan.

Co-decision making: Ideally, decisions about newborn care should be made jointly by carers and parents. This collaborative approach ensures that the child's well-being is always at the centre of concerns, while respecting the parents' autonomy.

Mediation: In some situations, despite the best of intentions, differences can arise between the medical team and the parents. Rather than allowing these tensions to escalate, mediation, whether by an external professional or a trained member of the team, can provide a space to explore these differences and find common ground.

Ongoing training: Respecting the beliefs and wishes of families requires specific skills. It is therefore crucial that neonatal healthcare professionals receive ongoing training in communication skills, cultural sensitivity and medical ethics.

Working with families in neonatology is a journey fraught with challenges, but also with profound rewards. By placing the relationship at the centre of care, and by fostering mutual respect and understanding, it is possible to transform the medical journey into an enriching and humane experience for everyone involved.

Chapter 9:
RESEARCH AND INNOVATION
IN NEONATOLOGY

The evolution of neonatal medicine : where do we stand?

Neonatal medicine, a medical speciality at the crossroads of technology, research and human compassion, has undergone major transformations in recent decades. From the simple care of newborn babies to cutting-edge medical interventions, it has constantly pushed back the boundaries of what is possible. But where do we stand today?

Modest beginnings: In the early years of neonatology, resources were limited. Premature babies were placed in rudimentary "incubators", often with little hope of survival for those born very early. Advances were mainly focused on nutrition and infection control.

The technological revolution: Over time, technology has made spectacular leaps forward. Advanced cardiac monitors, state-of-the-art ventilators, innovative oxygen therapy equipment and much more have made it possible to care for younger and younger babies, with ever-increasing survival rates.

Research and its benefits: Clinical studies have helped to improve care protocols. From the discovery of the benefits of pulmonary surfactant for premature babies to the importance of skin-to-skin care for neonatal well-being, research has constantly enriched our understanding and refined our interventions.

The holistic approach: Modern neonatology does not just look after the newborn's body. It recognises the importance of the environment, the family, sensory stimulation and human interaction. Today's neonatology units are less like sterile operating theatres and more like warm spaces conducive to development.

Genetics and personalised medicine: With advances in genetics, we are now able to identify certain conditions at an early stage and personalise treatments. This opens the way to more targeted interventions and, potentially, the prevention of certain complications.

Interdisciplinary collaboration: Today's neonatal care is the result of close collaboration between various professionals: paediatricians, nurses, physiotherapists, nutritionists, psychologists and many others. This integrated approach guarantees comprehensive care for newborn babies.

The challenges ahead: Although neonatology has made great strides, it faces new challenges, particularly in terms of medical ethics, healthcare costs, equitable access to care and the long-term management of premature babies.

Neonatal medicine is a reflection of our ability to marry science, technology and humanity. It is constantly evolving, learning from the past while looking to the future with optimism and ambition. At every stage, it reaffirms its deep commitment to those lives that are just beginning, those little sparks full of potential.

Participating in research : the importance of staying at the cutting edge

In the fast-paced world of medicine, research is the engine that drives innovation and shapes the future. Neonatology, like any other medical discipline, relies on continuous discoveries to improve care, increase survival rates and offer newborns a better quality of life. Participating in research is not just about acquiring new knowledge; it's essential to staying at the forefront of the field.

Discovering for better care: Every protocol, every treatment, every technique used in neonatology has its origin in research. It is thanks to rigorous clinical studies that we have a better understanding of the specific needs of premature babies, the mechanisms of neonatal diseases and the impact of interventions on long-term development.

Global impact: Participating in research means contributing to the global knowledge base. The results of a study can have repercussions far beyond national borders, influencing clinical practice throughout the world and offering new perspectives.

Professional recognition: For healthcare professionals, being active in research strengthens their credibility, positions them as opinion leaders and offers them opportunities for international collaboration.

Anticipating future challenges: By exploring the unknown terrain of neonatology, researchers can anticipate and respond to emerging challenges. Whether it's problems linked to new pathologies, complications arising from existing treatments or questions of medical ethics, research is paving the way for innovative solutions.

Fostering a culture of excellence: An institution or professional involved in research tends to foster a culture of excellence, constantly encouraging questioning, learning and improvement.

Interdisciplinary collaboration: Research in neonatology is not limited to paediatricians. It often involves multidisciplinary teams, from biochemists to psychologists, which enriches the overall understanding of neonatal issues.

Ethics and humanism: Being at the cutting edge of research also involves in-depth ethical reflection. Questions about medical intervention, consent or long-term implications require a holistic approach that combines science with humanity.

Research in neonatology is an exciting pursuit, combining hope, determination and ingenuity. By taking an active part in it, professionals not only broaden the horizons of their discipline but also ensure that the care offered to the smallest and most vulnerable among us is based on the latest and most solid knowledge.

Technological innovations and their impact on care

At the dawn of the 21st century, the medical landscape is constantly changing, largely thanks to technological innovations. Neonatology, the delicate field that cares for newborn babies, is no exception. Technological advances have not only pushed back the boundaries of what is medically possible, but have also transformed the way we care for even the most fragile babies.

Advanced   monitors : The arrival of sophisticated monitors has changed the game. Capable of monitoring a newborn's vital signs in real time, such as heart rate, oxygen saturation or blood pressure, they give medical teams a precise window on the child's state of health. This allows them to intervene proactively and avoid potential complications.

Improved ventilation: Modern ventilators are much better adapted to the needs of premature babies. With gentler ventilation modes, they minimise the risk of lung damage while ensuring optimal oxygenation.

Telemedicine: The ability to consult specialists remotely, access medical records in real time or monitor a baby's development after leaving the neonatal unit is revolutionising care. This ensures that, wherever they are, every baby can benefit from the necessary expertise.

Imaging equipment: Technologies such as ultrasound, MRI and advanced X-rays provide clear, detailed images, enabling more accurate diagnosis and better planning of interventions.

Specialised applications and software: Dedicated applications now enable more rigorous monitoring of care, nutrition, medication and developmental progress. They also facilitate communication between the various members of the care team.

Targeted therapies: Equipment such as phototherapy lamps to treat neonatal jaundice or cold therapy devices for certain brain lesions offer more effective and less invasive treatments.

Digital interaction with families: Camera systems allow parents to see their baby from a distance when they cannot be present. This strengthens the parent-child bond and provides essential emotional support.

Training and simulation: Thanks to hyper-realistic neonatal mannequins and simulation environments, medical staff can train to deal with various emergency scenarios, thereby improving the quality of care.

Technological innovations in neonatology have a profound impact: they improve not only survival rates and long-term outcomes for newborn babies, but also the experience of families and healthcare professionals. In this quest to provide the best possible start in life, technology is an invaluable ally, a tool that, when used wisely, can work wonders.

Chapter 10:
THE ROLE OF THE NURSE
IN THE EDUCATION OF PARENTS

Preparing parents for discharge: education and training

Leaving the neonatal unit is a moment of mixed joy and apprehension for many parents. After spending days, even weeks or months, watching their child being cared for by a team of professionals, the thought of taking over at home can seem overwhelming. This is where parental preparation, education and training become crucial.

Assessing specific needs: Every baby and every family is unique. Before planning training, it is essential to assess each family's specific needs, whether these relate to ongoing medical care, nutritional concerns or developmental needs.

Practical workshops: Practical sessions can be organised to teach parents essential skills such as how to feed their baby, how to give medicines, or how to perform therapeutic massages.

Awareness of vital signs: Parents can be trained to recognise their baby's vital signs, to understand what is normal and what may need medical attention.

Managing medical equipment: If the baby needs specific equipment at home, parents must be trained in its use and maintenance, whether it's a heart monitor, feeding pump or ventilation device.

Emotional support: Preparing for the birth is not just about physical care. Parents may need support to deal with anxiety, stress or the bereavement of a 'normal' birth experience.

Follow-up planning: Organising follow-up appointments, therapy sessions or support groups helps to ensure a smooth transition home and to continue supporting the family.

Resources and emergency contacts: Providing parents with a list of resources, including emergency numbers, home support contacts or parent support groups, can give them extra security.

Integrating brothers and sisters: It's also important to include brothers and sisters in the process. Preparing them for the arrival of their new brother or sister at home, with any special needs they may have, is crucial to ensuring family harmony.

Advice on the home environment: recommendations can be made to help prepare the home, whether it's accessibility improvements or advice on how to create a calm and stimulating environment for the baby.

The transition from hospital to home is a major step for the families of newborn babies who have required neonatal care. By equipping parents with the necessary skills, knowledge and confidence, healthcare professionals play an essential role in ensuring the baby's continued well-being and supporting the whole family in this new adventure.

Managing difficult situations: bereavements, bad news, etc.

Neonatology, for all its wonders and successes, also has its dark and painful moments. Nurses and other healthcare staff are often on the front line in these situations. They are confronted with parents' raw pain, grief, confusion and, sometimes, anger. Learning to navigate these moments with compassion, professionalism and resilience is crucial.

Empathetic communication: Delivering difficult news requires great sensitivity. This means not only choosing the right words, but also listening, recognising parents' emotions and offering immediate support.

Space for grief: Parents who have suffered a loss or received bad news need a space to process their emotions. Whether it's a quiet room away or support to help them get home, it's crucial to offer them this respite.

Offer resources: Whether it's bereavement support groups, therapies or recommended reading, directing parents to resources can help them manage their grief.

Ritual and memory: For parents who have lost a child, offering the opportunity to create memories, whether through photos, footprints or locks of hair, can be a valuable part of the grieving process.

Supporting the team: Nurses and doctors are also emotionally affected. Creating an environment where they can share their feelings, get psychological support or even take part in commemorative rituals strengthens the team's resilience.

Ongoing training: Training sessions on how to communicate bad news, the psychology of bereavement or crisis support can equip staff with the tools they need to manage these moments.

Recognising signs of distress: It's vital to be alert to signs of distress in parents - and among team members too. Recognising when someone needs help or time to recover is essential.

Inclusion of specialists: Bringing in psychologists, social workers or chaplains to accompany families and the team can offer additional support.

Taking a step back: Sometimes the best thing you can do is to take a step back. This might mean giving parents time alone with their baby, or allowing a member of the team to step away from the situation for a while.

Dark moments in neonatology are a reality that no one wants to face, but they are inevitable. With training, support and open communication, these situations can be managed with the dignity, respect and compassion they deserve.

Tools and resources for effective communication

Communication is a central pillar in neonatology. Clear, empathetic and precise communication is essential between carers, with parents, and sometimes even with the babies themselves. It can make the difference between a parent who feels supported and informed and one who feels lost and anxious. Here are some essential tools and resources to promote effective communication in neonatology.

Communication training: There are many programmes and workshops designed specifically to train healthcare professionals in empathetic and effective communication. These courses can cover topics such as delivering bad news, managing emotions or mediating in the event of disagreement.

Visual tools: Diagrams, computer graphics and scale models can help explain complex concepts or detail anatomy and physiology to parents, making the information more accessible.

Written guides: Brochures, leaflets and guides provide parents with a tangible resource that they can consult at their own pace. These materials can cover a wide range of topics, from understanding a specific illness to preparing for the return home.

Translation software: In care units where families speak a variety of languages, having access to reliable translation tools is invaluable in ensuring that each parent receives information in a language they understand.

Medical interpreters: Whenever possible, the use of interpreters trained in the medical field guarantees not only translation of the language, but also nuanced communication of medical terms.

Communication technology: Tablets, smartphones and computers can be used for telemedicine, enabling parents to communicate with doctors even from a distance, or to take part in multidisciplinary team meetings.

Regular   feedback: Organising regular feedback sessions with parents can help to identify areas where communication can be improved.

Logbooks and monitoring books: These enable ongoing communication between teams during changes of service. Parents can also write down any questions or concerns, ensuring two-way communication.

Support groups: These groups give parents the opportunity to share their experiences, ask questions and learn from each other, while being guided by a professional.

Active listening: This is perhaps the most important and yet most underestimated tool. Taking the time to really listen, without interruption, and to reflect what you hear can greatly improve the quality of communication.

By combining the right training, technological tools and tangible resources, neonatal staff can ensure that communication always remains at the heart of the care they provide, strengthening trust, understanding and partnership with the families they serve.

Chapter 11:
THE IMPORTANCE
OF MULTIDISCIPLINARITY

The role of each member
the neonatology medical team

Neonatology, far from being the work of a lone hero, is the result of intense collaboration between different healthcare professionals. Each member of this team plays a specific role, and it is the sum of their combined efforts that makes it possible to offer exceptional care to newborn babies and their families.

At the heart of this medical symphony is the **neonatologist**. An expert in the care of premature babies and newborns with pathologies, he is the conductor of the team, making crucial decisions about the diagnosis, treatment and follow-up of little patients.

Supporting the neonatologist in this mission, the **neonatal nurse** is the mainstay of day-to-day care. They are the eyes and ears of the department, constantly monitoring babies' vital signs, administering treatments and being the first responder in the event of an emergency. They also play a crucial role in supporting and educating parents, guiding them through the ocean of emotions and uncertainties that a stay in the neonatal unit represents.

The **physiotherapist** then intervenes, helping newborn babies to develop their lung function and overcome any respiratory complications. Using specialised techniques, he or she stimulates and strengthens their young lungs, preparing them for life outside the incubator.

Although less visible, the **pharmacist** plays an equally essential role. As experts in medicines, they ensure that every baby receives the right medicine, in the right dose, at the right time. Working in partnership with the neonatologist, they ensure that the best possible treatment is given, tailored to each individual situation.

The **psychologist** is the team's emotional beacon. She provides support and advice to parents dealing with anxiety, stress or grief, while also offering a sympathetic ear to members of the medical team, who are often faced with emotionally charged situations.

Finally, the **dietician** ensures that each baby receives the nutrition adapted to its specific needs. In collaboration with the nurse, they draw up nutritional plans to promote the growth and health of newborn babies.

This team, although made up of individuals with varied skills, works towards a common goal: ensuring the well-being and health of the smallest and most vulnerable among us. And it is this collaboration, this unity of vision, that makes neonatology such a special and vital part of the medical world.

How to work efficiently with various specialists

Interprofessional collaboration is at the heart of modern medicine. The increasing complexity of care requires seamless coordination between different specialists to ensure the best possible outcome for the patient. Here are some tips on how to work effectively with different specialists:

Understanding the role of each specialist: Before you can work in tandem with other professionals, it's essential to understand their area of expertise, their responsibilities and the value they bring to the team.

Open and respectful communication: It is crucial to encourage open dialogue, avoiding jargon wherever possible and listening actively. Mutual respect also facilitates productive communication.

Organise regular meetings: Regular meetings ensure that everyone is on the same wavelength regarding the care plan, patient updates and any concerns.

Use collaborative tools: From electronic medical records to specialist communication applications, technological tools can help keep everyone informed in real time.

Promoting interdisciplinary training: When specialists understand the basics of other fields, they can better anticipate the needs of the team and facilitate comprehensive patient care.

Clarify responsibilities: Avoid confusion by clearly establishing who is responsible for what. This reduces the risk of duplication or neglect of care.

Giving and receiving feedback: An interprofessional team can always improve. By encouraging constructive feedback, team members can continually adapt and improve.

Cultivating a team spirit: Team-building activities and moments of shared relaxation can strengthen the bonds between team members and facilitate better collaboration.

Being flexible: Every patient is unique, and sometimes the established plan needs to be adjusted. The ability to adapt quickly to new information or changing situations is essential.

Putting the patient first: Beyond areas of expertise, egos and professional differences, the patient's well-being must always remain the central priority. This helps to keep the team focused and united in its objective.

Working effectively with different specialists requires openness, respect, clear communication and a commitment to the patient's well-being. It is by joining forces that specialists can offer holistic and optimised care.

Chapter 12:
NUTRITIONAL ASPECTS
IN NEONATOLOGY

The importance of nutrition
for newborn babies

The neonatal period is a critical window in an individual's life. In these first few weeks of life, the body undergoes rapid and fundamental transformations that will lay the foundations for future health. At the heart of these changes lies nutrition. The nutritional needs of newborn babies are specific, intense and crucial to their healthy growth and development.

- **Rapid growth :** Newborn babies, particularly premature ones, undergo exponential growth. Caloric and nutritional requirements during this period are therefore proportionately higher than for any other stage of life. Adequate nutrition ensures healthy growth of bones, muscles and organs.
- **Brain development:** The first few months of life are essential for brain development. Fatty acids such as omega-3 are vital for the formation of neurons and synapses. Optimal nutritional intake has a positive influence on future cognitive and emotional abilities.
- **Immune system:** A newborn baby's immune system is still developing. Colostrum, the first form of breast milk, is rich in antibodies that protect the baby from infection. What's more, proper nutrition strengthens the intestinal barrier, reducing the risk of infection.
- **Metabolism:** Adequate nutrition during the neonatal period can have a lasting impact on an individual's metabolism. It influences weight regulation, glucose tolerance and other metabolic aspects throughout life.

Motor development: Nutrition influences muscle strength and coordination. Adequate protein and micronutrient intake is essential for motor development.

Disease prevention: Nutritional deficiencies at this early stage can predispose to chronic illnesses in adulthood, such as diabetes, hypertension and certain heart diseases.

Hormone regulation: Hormones play a key role in growth and development. Nutrition influences the production and regulation of these hormones.

Emotional well-being: Although less obvious, there is a link between nutrition and mood. Nutritional imbalances can affect behaviour and mood, even in infants.

Good digestion: A healthy digestive system starts with good nutrition. It ensures healthy intestinal flora, reducing the risk of colic, constipation and other digestive disorders.

The role of nutrition for newborn babies is therefore deeply rooted in every aspect of their development and health. By ensuring optimal nutrition from the very first days of life, we are laying the foundations for a healthy and fulfilling life. It's not just an act of feeding; it's an act of love, foresight and commitment to a child's future.

Different feeding methods: breastfeeding, enteral feeding, parenteral feeding, etc.

The way in which a newborn baby is fed depends on its state of health, its ability to suckle, its nutritional needs and sometimes the parents' choices. Here's an exploration of the different feeding methods that can be used depending on the situation.

Breastfeeding:

Natural and physiological: Breastfeeding is the most natural and recommended method of feeding newborn babies. Breast milk is rich in nutrients, antibodies and other beneficial factors that promote growth, protection and development.

Benefits: In addition to its nutritional advantages, breastfeeding strengthens the bond between mother and child, stimulates milk production and reduces the risk of certain illnesses for both mother and child.

Formula milk: For mothers who cannot or do not wish to breastfeed, formula milk is an alternative. It is designed to be as close as possible to the composition of breast milk.

Enteral feeding :

Introduction: Enteral feeding is used for babies who cannot suck or swallow effectively but whose digestive system is functioning normally.

Nasogastric tube: A thin tube is inserted through the nose, passes through the oesophagus and ends in the stomach. It allows milk to be administered directly into the stomach.

Orogastric tube: Similar to the nasogastric tube, this tube is inserted through the mouth.

Naso-intestinal tube: This tube goes further than the stomach, ending in the small intestine, and is generally used when the stomach cannot process food properly.

Parenteral nutrition :

Introduction: Parenteral nutrition is used when a baby's digestive system cannot or should not be used. Nutrients are administered directly into the bloodstream.

Total parenteral nutrition (TPN): When all nutritional needs are covered by this method.

Partial parenteral nutrition: Used to supplement enteral nutrition.

Route of administration: Nutrients are generally administered via a central or peripheral venous catheter.

Each of these methods has its own advantages, risks and indications. The choice often depends on the baby's clinical condition, nutritional needs and the ability of parents and carers to manage the chosen method. What all these methods have in common is their ultimate goal: to ensure that every newborn baby receives the nutrition they need to grow and develop in good health. Close collaboration between health professionals, parents and carers is essential if this mission is to be achieved.

Common nutritional challenges and solutions

Nutrition plays an essential role in the healthy development of a newborn baby, particularly in the neonatal unit where babies may have specific needs due to premature birth or medical conditions. Understanding common nutritional challenges and knowing how to respond to them is vital for care staff.

Insufficient weight gain :

Challenge: Newborn babies, especially premature ones, can have difficulty gaining weight.

Solution: Increase the calorie density of milk or formula, closely monitor intake and growth, and consult a paediatric nutritionist for specific recommendations.

- Food intolerance :

  Challenge: Signs include vomiting, diarrhoea, bloating and abnormal stools.

  Solution: Reduce or space out intakes, use specialised formulas, watch out for signs of allergies or intolerances.

- Necrotizing enterocolitis (NEC) :

  Challenge: This is a serious intestinal disease that can occur in premature babies.

  Solution: Use breast milk, which appears to reduce the risk, monitor closely for signs of NEC, and stop feeding if symptoms appear, while starting appropriate medical treatment.

- Sucking and swallowing difficulties :

  Challenge: Premature babies may not yet have developed the reflexes needed to suck and swallow effectively.

  Solution: Use breastfeeding support techniques, specialised teats, or consider alternative feeding methods such as tubes.

- Hypoglycaemia :

  Challenge: Some babies can have low blood sugar levels after birth.

  Solution: Regular monitoring of blood glucose levels, rapid intake of glucose or milk and, in severe cases, use of intravenous glucose solutions.

- Vitamin and mineral deficiencies :

  Challenge: Premature babies may have increased requirements for certain vitamins and minerals.

  Solution: Supplementation with specific vitamins and minerals as recommended, and regular monitoring of blood levels.

Hyperbilirubinemia or jaundice:

  Challenge: It is caused by an excess of bilirubin in the blood, often visible as a yellow discolouration of the skin.

  Solution: Increase dietary intake to promote bilirubin excretion, and use phototherapy if necessary.

Nutritional challenges in neonatology require an individualised, multidisciplinary approach, involving paediatricians, nutritionists, nurses and parents. A thorough understanding of these challenges and early intervention can make a significant difference to the long-term health and development of the newborn.

Chapter 13:
SPECIFIC PHARMACOLOGY
NEONATOLOGY

Commonly used medicines and their indications

Pharmacotherapy in neonatology is complex because of the unique physiology of newborn babies, particularly premature babies. Here is a non-exhaustive list of commonly used drugs and their main indications.

Pulmonary surfactant :
> **Indication:** Treatment of respiratory distress in premature babies.
> **Mechanism:** Replaces the lungs' natural surfactant, which can be lacking in premature babies.

Caffeine :
> **Indication:** Apnoea in premature babies.
> **Mechanism:** Stimulates the respiratory centre to reduce apnoea episodes.

Antibiotics (such as ampicillin and gentamicin):
> **Indication:** Suspected or confirmed infections.
> **Mechanism:** Fight against pathogenic bacteria.

Furosemide :
> **Indication:** Pulmonary oedema or heart failure.
> **Mechanism:** Diuretic which increases renal excretion of water and electrolytes.

Dopamine, Dobutamine :
> **Indication:** Heart failure or shock.

Mechanism: Increases the force of cardiac contraction and/or blood pressure.

Indomethacin, Ibuprofen :

Indication: Closure of persistent ductus arteriosus.

Mechanism: Inhibits prostaglandin, promoting canal closure.

Vitamin K :

Indication: Prophylaxis of haemorrhagic disease in newborns.

Mechanism: Essential for blood coagulation.

Erythropoietin :

Indication: Anemia of prematurity.

Mechanism: Stimulates the production of red blood cells.

Acyclovir :

Indication: Herpes simplex infections.

Mechanism: Antiviral.

Phenobarbital, levetiracetam :

Indication: Epileptic seizures.

Mechanism: anti-epileptic drugs.

Ranitidine, Omeprazole :

Indication: Gastro-oesophageal reflux disease or ulcers.

Mechanism: Reduces gastric acid production.

It is important to note that the pharmacokinetics and pharmacodynamics of medicines vary considerably in newborns, and particularly in premature babies. As a result, doses, indications and side effects may differ from those of older children or adults. Always consult appropriate specialist resources when prescribing or administering medicines to this population.

Dosage, administration and monitoring of side effects

In neonatology, the correct administration of medicines is crucial, given the vulnerability of patients. Here's a fluid exploration of these key elements.

The Art of Dosage
Every millilitre counts in neonatology. Dosage is generally based on the infant's weight, often in mg/kg. This calculation is essential, because a simple deviation can have major consequences. The baby's physiological development must also be taken into account, as the metabolism, excretion and distribution of drugs vary according to gestational and postnatal age.

Administration: Surgical Precision
There are many routes of administration in neonatology: oral, intravenous, intra-arterial, subcutaneous, intramuscular, intrathecal and more. Each route has its own specific features:

- **Oral:** Often preferred for its simplicity, but absorption capacity may vary in premature babies.
- **Intravenous:** Provides rapid onset of action, but requires extra monitoring of the injection site to prevent infection.

Monitoring side effects: a sharp eye
Even with impeccable dosing, side effects are always possible. Some signs are obvious, such as a skin rash, while others, such as kidney failure, require more detailed analysis. Observation is the key word. Any change in behaviour, breathing, skin colour or even the consistency of stools can be a clue.

But monitoring does not stop there. Regular check-ups, such as blood tests, ultrasounds and X-rays, may be necessary to detect any complications.

Collaboration: the key to safety

Medication safety is a shared responsibility. Pharmacists, doctors and nurses need to work closely together to ensure the correct treatment is given. Errors are human, but in neonatology, the margins for error are slim. Double or triple checking of doses is often practised.

Parent education

Educating parents is also crucial. They need to understand why a drug is being administered, what the expected effects are, and what warning signs they should look out for at home, particularly if the baby has been discharged from the care unit.

Neonatology is a field where every detail counts. Dosage, administration and monitoring are essential pillars of drug management. It's a delicate ballet, where science meets art, with the sole aim of ensuring the well-being of the newborn.

Specific pharmacokinetics in neonates

The newborn, and in particular the premature baby, is a unique physiological entity with specific characteristics that have a profound influence on the pharmacokinetics of medicines. Let's dive seamlessly into this fascinating world of medicines and babies.

A Body in Constant Change

At the beginning of life, everything is in motion. Organs, systems, circulation... all evolve at dizzying speed. These changes have an impact on the way medicines are absorbed, distributed, metabolised and excreted.

Absorption: Tailor-made input

The route of administration has a major influence on absorption. For example, the skin of a premature baby is thinner and less mature, making the penetration of drugs administered transdermally more unpredictable. Reduced gastric acidity in newborns also influences the absorption of drugs administered orally.

Distribution: Un Voyage Particulier

The proportions of water and fat in the body of a newborn differ from those of an adult. With a higher proportion of water, water-soluble drugs may have a larger volume of distribution. In addition, as the carrier protein system is still immature, this can affect the binding of drugs to plasma proteins, making more drugs available for action.

Metabolism: A Lapping Factory

The liver is the main organ for drug metabolism. In newborns, particularly premature babies, the liver is immature. Certain enzyme systems, such as cytochrome P450, may not be fully functional. This can slow down the metabolism of certain drugs and increase their duration of action or side effects.

Excretion: a gentle but slow system

The kidneys are the main excretory organs. But like the liver, the kidneys of newborn babies are immature. Their capacity to filter, reabsorb and secrete can be reduced, influencing the length of time a drug remains in the system.

The key: Necessary individualisation

All these specific features mean that the same medicine can act differently from one baby to the next. This is why neonatal pharmacokinetics require individualisation of doses, careful monitoring and close collaboration between the various members of the medical team.

Understanding the specific pharmacokinetics of newborn babies is essential if we are to ensure that medicines are administered safely and effectively. It's a challenge, certainly, but one that lies at the heart of ensuring a healthy future for these fragile little lives.

Chapter 14:
COMPLEMENTARY THERAPIES AND ALTERNATIVES

Non-conventional approaches neonatology: music therapy, therapeutic touch

At the heart of the medical world, where technology and science dominate, neonatology stands out for its ability to recognise the importance of humanity and intuition. In addition to advanced medical care, the world of newborn care has gradually incorporated unconventional therapies to improve the quality of care. Let's delve into the gentle world of music therapy and therapeutic touch.

Music therapy: the gentle melody of well-being

Music, in all its forms, has long been recognised for its therapeutic properties. In neonatology, music therapy offers a gentle oasis in a sometimes noisy and stressful environment.

- **Physiological impact**: Studies have shown that soft music can stabilise heart rate, improve oxygen saturation and reduce stress levels in premature babies.
- **Neurological stimulation**: Music helps the brain to mature, by stimulating the regions associated with listening and auditory processing.
- **Parent-child bonding**: Singing or playing music for your baby can help strengthen the emotional bond, especially when a parent feels helpless in the face of medical challenges.

Therapeutic touch: The Power of the Caring Hand

Touch is one of the first senses to develop in utero. In

neonatology, therapeutic touch goes beyond simple physical contact.

Baby massage: Gentle massages can help regulate bodily functions, improve digestion and promote sleep. For parents, massaging their baby can be a way of being active in caring for them and establishing a bond.

Skin-to-skin or kangaroo method: This method, which involves placing the naked baby against a parent's chest, can have incredible effects on thermal regulation, cardiac and respiratory stabilisation and breastfeeding.

Each of these unconventional approaches brings an extra dimension to neonatal care. They recognise that, as well as being fragile beings in need of medical care, newborns are also sensitive human beings, responding to love, touch and music. In this delicate dance of life, the fusion of science and sensitivity creates a symphony of holistic care for our smallest patients.

Studies and associated benefits

When it comes to caring for newborn babies, particularly premature babies, the importance of evidence-based studies is indisputable. It is through this scientific lens that non-conventional approaches, such as music therapy and therapeutic touch, reveal their remarkable benefits, supporting the healing, growth and development of little neonatal patients. Read on to discover the studies and benefits associated with these alternative therapeutic practices.

Studies on Music Therapy

Clinical research: Research shows that music, specifically selected and administered, can positively influence the physiology of newborns. Studies have shown significant improvements in the stability of vital signs, waking and sleeping behaviour, and feeding ability.

Proven benefits: As well as the physiological benefits, music therapy can also contribute to neurological development, stimulating the auditory pathways and strengthening the parent-child connection.

Studies on Therapeutic Touch

Scientific evidence: Therapeutic touch, particularly massage and skin-to-skin contact, is widely studied. Babies who benefit from this intervention show improvements in weight gain, temperature regulation and a reduction in stress and pain.

Proven benefits: The benefits also extend to the mental health of parents, who experience less stress and anxiety and a stronger emotional bond with their baby.

Studies on other complementary approaches

Scientific exploration: Other complementary therapies, such as light therapy and animal therapy, are currently being explored. Although the data is still emerging, preliminary results are promising.

Potential benefits: These therapies have the potential to improve mood, reduce anxiety and contribute to the overall well-being of newborns and their families.

The assimilation of non-conventional approaches in neonatal care is firmly based on solid scientific studies and evidence. These complementary methods, carefully and respectfully integrated into conventional care, enrich the care experience of newborns and their families, offering a holistic and harmonious healing pathway.

How to integrate them safely

In neonatology, safety is paramount. Introducing unconventional therapies requires a well thought-out approach, to ensure the well-being of newborns while maximising the potential benefits of these practices. Here's how to incorporate them safely.

Preliminary assessment

Medical check-up: Before any intervention, a full assessment of the newborn's state of health is essential. Certain medical conditions may make therapy inappropriate or require adjustments.

Background knowledge: It is crucial to understand the baby's background, previous reactions to various stimuli, and any other relevant information that may influence how he or she responds to therapy.

Professional Training

Certification and training: Make sure practitioners are certified and trained in the specific therapy they offer. For example, a qualified music therapist will have in-depth knowledge of how to use music therapeutically with newborns.

Continuing education: Medicine is constantly evolving, as are complementary therapies. It is therefore essential that professionals undergo regular training to keep up to date.

Protocols and Guidelines

Developing protocols: Establish clear protocols for each therapy. This includes indications, contraindications, duration, frequency and any other relevant details.

Follow-up and monitoring: As with traditional medical care, continuous monitoring during and after therapy is crucial. This allows any signs of stress or negative reactions to be identified quickly.

Collaboration and Communication

Interprofessional communication: Therapists need to work closely with the medical team. A regular exchange of information ensures that everyone is aware of progress, concerns or changes in the care plan.

Informing parents: Parents must be fully informed of what each therapy involves, the potential benefits, possible risks and what they can expect. Their informed consent is vital.

Revaluation and adjustments

Feedback: After each session, take a moment to assess how the baby has responded. This will help refine future sessions to maximise the benefits.

Flexibility: Be prepared to adapt or interrupt a therapy if it does not seem to be beneficial or if it causes any distress.

The safe integration of non-conventional approaches into neonatal care requires careful planning, specialist training, constant communication and ongoing evaluation. With these elements in place, these therapies can offer a valuable addition to the range of care available to newborns and their families.

Chapter 15:
THE IMPORTANCE OF CARE
FAMILY-CENTRED

Involvement of parents
in the care of their child

In the cosy but sometimes frightening world of the neonatal unit, parents play an essential role, acting as emotional and physical pillars for their newborn. While health professionals are busy working around incubators, monitors and other medical equipment, parents are often faced with a host of emotions: anxiety, hope, guilt and the desire to feel useful. In this context, the active involvement of parents in their child's care is not only beneficial for the baby, but also for themselves.

The benefits of parental involvement
When parents are actively involved in care, there are a number of benefits:

Strengthening the emotional bond: Skin-to-skin contact, also known as "kangarooing", promotes closeness and bonding between baby and parents. This interaction stimulates the production of oxytocin, the attachment hormone.

Stimulation of development: Parent-child interaction can help to improve the baby's temperature regulation, stabilise the heart rate and even promote better growth.

Stress reduction: For babies, feeling the reassuring presence of their parents can reduce stress levels. And for parents, feeling active and useful can help reduce anxiety and feelings of helplessness.

Simple but precious gestures

Feeding: Whether through breastfeeding or bottle-feeding, feeding your baby is an intimate moment of connection.

Bathing: Learning to bathe a premature or sick newborn can be intimidating, but it's a skill that parents can master with the support of the medical team.

Singing and talking: Talking, singing or simply whispering in your baby's ear can reassure them and strengthen the parent-child bond.

A partnership with the medical team

Training and education: Nurses and doctors can teach parents the basics of neonatal care, familiarising them with equipment and routines.

Involvement in decision-making: Involving parents in the decision-making process concerning their child's care reinforces their central role in the care team.

Emotional support: Recognising and validating parents' emotions, listening to them and offering them psychological support is crucial to their well-being.

Parents' involvement in their child's care in the neonatal unit transcends the simple act of "caring". It forges a triangle of love, dedication and science, in which each member - the baby, the parents and the medical team - plays an irreplaceable role in ensuring the best possible start to the life of this new little being.

Holistic approach : consider the newborn in the family environment

The holistic approach in neonatology is not limited to treating the symptoms or medical conditions of the newborn. It takes into account the child as a whole, integrating his or her physical, emotional, social and even spiritual environment. In this respect, the family plays a vital role. Recognising the importance of this family environment and actively including it in the care process helps to create a harmonious balance between the infant's medical needs and his or her overall well-being.

The child at the heart of a network of interactions
Each newborn is a unique entity, but they are also the product of a history, a culture and a family network. Their interactions with those closest to them, even at such a tender age, shape their experience of the world.

- **Emotional connection**: The first days and weeks of a baby's life are crucial for establishing an emotional bond with his parents. This emotional bond serves as the foundation for the baby's future emotional development.
- **Cultural transmission**: Rituals, songs, stories and cultural practices passed on by the family play a decisive role in anchoring a child's culture and identity.

The vital role of the family
Involving the family in the care process goes far beyond simply providing comfort:

- **Understanding needs**: Parents, in particular, are often best placed to recognise the subtle signs of their baby's comfort or discomfort.
- **Continuity of care**: At home, family members will continue to provide the child's day-to-day care.

Preparing and educating them is therefore essential for a smooth transition.

Psychological support: Relatives can offer invaluable emotional support, both for the baby and for other family members, at times of stress or uncertainty.

Harmonisation with the medical team

Open communication: A relationship of trust between the medical team and the family is essential to ensure optimal care. Mutual understanding of concerns, hopes and fears facilitates appropriate care.

Education and training: Providing families with the necessary tools and knowledge strengthens their ability to play an active role in their child's care.

The holistic approach to neonatology recognises that each baby is more than a sum of medical symptoms to be treated. He or she is a complex human being, embedded in a rich web of interactions and relationships. By placing the newborn at the centre of a loving family environment and in harmony with the medical team, we maximise his or her chances of a harmonious and fulfilling development.

Chapter 16:
SAFETY IN NEONATOLOGY

Avoiding medical errors and guarantee patient safety

In the high-stakes world of medicine, ensuring patient safety is an absolute priority. This task takes on even greater importance in neonatology, where vulnerable and delicate patients require unfailing attention and precision. Avoiding medical errors relies not only on clinical expertise, but also on an institutional culture, effective communication and ongoing training.

Every intervention, every drug administered and every decision taken in the neonatal unit has a potentially lasting impact on a newborn's well-being. In this intense atmosphere, a simple distraction can lead to mistakes. But how can we ensure that every action taken is the right one?

First and foremost, a hospital culture focused on safety is essential. Teams need to adopt a proactive approach, anticipating risks and putting clear protocols in place. These protocols must be regularly reviewed and updated to reflect current best practice.

Secondly, communication plays a decisive role. Incorrect transmission of information, whether about a patient's condition, a drug dosage or a procedure to be followed, can have devastating consequences. Teams therefore need to ensure that every piece of information is clear, accurate and confirmed by all parties involved. Modern technologies, such as electronic medical records, can be invaluable allies in this quest for accuracy.

Continuing education is also crucial. Medicine is evolving rapidly, and what was considered best practice a few years ago may no longer be so today. Neonatal professionals must therefore be committed to continuous learning, familiarising themselves with the latest advances and techniques to ensure the best possible care.

Finally, it is vital to consider the human element behind the professional. Fatigue, stress or burnout can affect performance and decision-making. Taking care of medical teams, allowing them sufficient time to rest and offering them emotional support also means guaranteeing patient safety.

Ensuring the safety of the youngest among us is no simple task. It requires dedication, rigour and constant questioning. But by always putting the well-being of the newborn at the centre of our concerns, cultivating a culture of excellence and investing in the training and well-being of our professionals, we can minimise mistakes and give every child the safest possible start in life.

The importance of reporting and safety culture

In the vast world of medicine, where every action can affect a patient's life, a safety culture is of paramount importance. This culture cannot be built overnight, but it is based on one fundamental pillar: reporting. This is how healthcare establishments identify risks, learn from their mistakes and, ultimately, offer safer care.

Far from being an admission of weakness, the act of reporting is a courageous and essential step. In an ideal world, medical errors would not exist. However, the reality is more complex. Medical care is part of a chain of actions and decisions involving many players. Errors can occur at any point in this chain. Whistleblowing is a way of bringing these failings to light, not to punish, but to understand and rectify.

An organisation with a strong safety culture will actively encourage reporting. Teams see it as a learning opportunity rather than a threat. Every incident reported is an opportunity for improvement, a wake-up call to rethink protocols, step up training or adopt new tools. Without this feedback, the same errors could be repeated indefinitely, putting patients at risk and undermining public confidence in the healthcare system.

In addition, reporting feeds into a valuable database, contributing to a broader view of trends, emerging risks and areas requiring special attention. This macroscopic perspective helps to guide healthcare policies, allocate resources more effectively and anticipate future challenges.

But for this culture to flourish, we need to create an environment where staff feel safe to report, without fear of negative repercussions. This requires committed management, clear and accessible reporting mechanisms and guarantees of non-retaliation.

Finally, the culture of safety, reinforced by the systematic practice of reporting, offers a more human vision of medicine. It recognises that healthcare professionals, however dedicated and competent they may be, are human and therefore prone to error. Rather than stigmatising these errors, it seeks to learn from them, so that every patient benefits from increasingly safe, effective and caring care.

Preventive measures and protocols in place

At the heart of neonatal care, where patients are among the most vulnerable, the implementation of preventive measures and rigorous protocols is essential to guarantee their safety and well-being. These protocols are intended both as safeguards against potential errors and as guides to optimal care.

Ongoing training: Medicine is constantly evolving. Neonatal carers therefore need regular training to keep them up to date with the latest advances and best practice. Simulations, workshops and conferences are organised to ensure that skills are constantly upgraded.

Checklists and cross-checks: To ensure that crucial steps are not forgotten, checklists are used, particularly for complex procedures. These checklists encourage consistency and limit errors of omission.

Disinfection protocols: Newborn babies have immature immune systems. Strict sterilisation and disinfection protocols are therefore essential to prevent nosocomial infections.

Patient identification: Measures are taken to ensure that each baby is correctly identified, with identification bracelets and mother-child matching systems, minimising the risk of errors.

Medication and infusions: Protocols ensure that the medicines administered are not only the right ones, but also at the right dose. Double checking, where two professionals check independently, is commonly used.

Infant feeding: There are precise guidelines for the preparation and administration of breast milk or infant formula, with regular checks to avoid any risk of contamination.

102

Equipment safety: Equipment such as incubators, ventilators and cardiac monitors undergo regular checks and maintenance to ensure that they are working properly.

Transfer protocol: The transfer of a newborn baby, whether within the hospital or to another establishment, is surrounded by numerous precautions to guarantee its safety during the transfer.

Emotional support: Care is not limited to the physical dimension. Emotional support protocols are also put in place for parents faced with the distress of seeing their child in the neonatal unit.

Morbidity and mortality reviews: These regular meetings enable the team to discuss complex cases, complications or deaths that have occurred, with a view to continuous improvement.

Aware of its responsibilities, the neonatal unit relies on a multitude of protocols to guarantee the highest possible level of care. These preventive measures, while requiring constant vigilance, are the foundation on which the trust of families and the reputation for excellence of neonatal units are built.

Chapter 17:
SIMULATION AND PRACTICAL TRAINING

The importance of training by simulation in neonatology

In the delicate field of neonatology, every gesture counts, every second can be crucial, and the ability to act promptly and effectively is an essential prerequisite. This is where simulation training comes in, a teaching method that has revolutionised the way healthcare professionals prepare to manage complex situations in neonatology.

Learning in a safe environment: Simulation provides a space where errors do not have real consequences, allowing learners to practise without risk. It's a training ground where professionals can familiarise themselves with rare or critical situations without putting a patient's life at risk.

Reproduction of real-life scenarios: Thanks to sophisticated mannequins and high-tech simulation environments, it is possible to faithfully reproduce clinical scenarios ranging from respiratory distress to neonatal resuscitation. This provides an immersive experience that is difficult to match by other teaching methods.

Reinforcing technical skills: Simulation helps to refine technical skills, whether it's intubating a premature baby, inserting a venous line or using equipment correctly.

Developing non-technical skills: Beyond purely technical skills, simulation emphasises equally vital skills such as communication, teamwork, decision-making and stress management.

- **Evaluation and feedback:** After each simulation, a debriefing phase is essential. It provides an opportunity to discuss what went well, areas for improvement and lessons to be learned. This direct feedback is invaluable for learning and consolidating skills.
- **Preparing for rare situations:** Certain complications in neonatology are rare, but when they do arise, they require rapid and competent action. Simulation allows us to prepare for these eventualities, even if they are never encountered in real-life practice.
- **Promoting a safety culture:** By reproducing scenarios that incorporate common mistakes, simulation helps to make professionals aware of potential pitfalls, thereby promoting a proactive safety culture.
- **Interdisciplinarity:** simulation sessions can bring together different professions, from doctors to nurses to physiotherapists, fostering a better understanding of each other's roles and reinforcing team spirit.
- **Regular updating:** As medicine evolves, simulation scenarios can be adapted to reflect changes in practices, guidelines or recommendations.

Simulation-based training in neonatology is much more than just a teaching tool: it is a central pillar of modern training, ensuring that professionals are ready to provide the highest quality care to neonatal patients and their families. In a specialty where the margins for error are slim, this preparation is invaluable.

Common scenarios and how they prepare you for clinical reality

Neonatology simulation uses carefully developed scenarios to mimic common clinical situations. These scenarios play a vital role in preparing healthcare professionals for the reality of the field. Here are some common examples and how they provide training in clinical reality:

Respiratory distress at birth :

Scenario: A newborn shows signs of respiratory distress immediately after delivery.

Learning: This scenario prepares staff to quickly identify symptoms, initiate mask ventilation and even perform intubation if necessary. It emphasises effective communication between team members and the importance of rapid stabilisation.

Neonatal resuscitation :

Scenario: A newborn baby does not breathe and has no detectable heart rhythm after birth.

Learning: This exercise teaches the stages of neonatal cardiopulmonary resuscitation, team coordination and the appropriate use of drugs and equipment.

Insertion of an umbilical vein :

Scenario: A premature baby requires urgent administration of medication and intravenous access.

Learning: Participants learn how to insert an umbilical vein correctly, a delicate but essential skill in neonatology.

Suspected meningeal haemorrhage :

Scenario: A newborn presents with neurological symptoms and requires a lumbar puncture.

Learning: Carers practise carrying out this technical procedure in calm, safe conditions, while managing the parents' anxiety.

Communicating bad news:

Scenario: Parents need to be informed of a serious anomaly or complication concerning their child.

Learning points: This scenario, often played out with actors playing the role of parents, teaches empathetic and clear communication skills.

Transfer of a critical patient :

Scenario: A newborn requires urgent transfer to a specialist unit.

Learning: Staff learn how to stabilise and prepare infants for transport while communicating effectively with transport teams and reception units.

Managing an epidemic in a unit :

Scenario: Several newborn babies develop a nosocomial infection.

Learning: Carers practise identifying the source, implementing isolation measures and communicating with parents and other services.

These scenarios, among many others, immerse professionals in situations they are likely to encounter in their careers. By experiencing them in a controlled environment, they gain in confidence and competence, ready to face clinical reality with confidence and expertise.

Feedback, debriefing and continuous improvement

The world of neonatology is complex, delicate and constantly evolving. Every intervention, every action, every decision can have huge repercussions. In this context, the culture of feedback, debriefing and continuous improvement is of paramount importance. This is the path to excellence, ensuring that babies receive the best possible care.

The importance of feedback :

Instantaneity: Immediate feedback after a procedure or interaction can help reinforce good practice or quickly correct an error. In neonatology, where every second counts, this speed is essential.

Constructiveness: The aim of good feedback is not to criticise, but to build. It's about sharing observations, suggestions and encouragement to help each team member improve.

The power of debriefing :

Collective reflection: After a critical situation, a debriefing enables the team to come together, discuss the events, understand what went well and identify areas for improvement.

Emotional learning: In neonatology, emotions can be intense. Debriefing provides a space to process these emotions, offering support and understanding.

Commitment to continuous improvement:

Updating skills: Medicine is constantly evolving. It is essential that professionals keep abreast of the latest research, techniques and recommendations.

Adapting protocols: Based on feedback, protocols can be adapted to ensure safer and more effective care.

Incorporating technologies : With the emergence of new technologies, it is crucial to adapt to maximise their potential to serve patients.

Safety   culture :

Reporting incidents: Rather than punishing mistakes, we need to see them as learning opportunities. If reported quickly, these mistakes can lead to major improvements.

Transparency: A culture where every member feels safe to share their concerns, doubts and mistakes is essential for continuous improvement.

Neonatology is an area where the margin for error is minimal and where excellence is expected. Feedback, debriefing and continuous improvement are not simply 'add-ons' to practice - they are at the very heart of quality care. Every member of the team, from nurses to paediatricians, has a collective responsibility to embrace these principles to ensure that every baby has the best chance of a healthy start in life.

Chapter 18:
LEAVING THE UNIT
NEONATOLOGY AND FOLLOW-UP

Preparing for the trip :
assessment and education of parents

When a newborn's vital signs stabilise and their state of health improves, the prospect of taking them home is on the horizon. Yet this stage, eagerly awaited by many parents, is also fraught with apprehension. At the heart of this transition, the neonatal nurse plays a crucial role in ensuring that the discharge from hospital goes smoothly. Preparing for this stage is twofold: it involves both the medical assessment of the child and the education of the parents.

- Newborn assessment :
  - **Clinical stability: Above** all, it is vital to ensure that the newborn is stable enough to leave the controlled environment of the neonatal unit. This involves regular checks of vital signs, the ability to maintain body temperature and regular weight gain.
  - **Final examinations:** Screening tests, such as the Guthrie test, are carried out to identify any metabolic or genetic abnormalities.
  - **Vaccinations:** Depending on your age and the length of your stay in hospital, some vaccinations may be necessary before discharge.
- Parent education :
  - **Basic care:** Although some parents already have children of their own, the specific care to be given to a premature baby or a newborn

who has required a stay in neonatology is crucial. They need to be trained in essential procedures such as bathing, changing nappies and taking temperatures.

Feeding: Parents need to be comfortable with the feeding method they choose, whether breast-feeding, bottle-feeding or, in some cases, enteral feeding.

Warning signs: Recognising the signs of distress in their child is vital. Parents need to know when to seek help and not hesitate if in doubt.

Medical appointments: Post-hospital follow-ups are essential, including consultations with the paediatrician, physiotherapists or specialists if necessary.

Emotional support :

Sharing emotions: Leaving hospital is a mixture of excitement and anxiety. The nurse is there to reassure, listen and guide parents through this new stage.

External resources: It's essential to make parents aware of the associations, support groups and specialist professionals who can help them in the weeks and months ahead.

Preparing for discharge from hospital is a fundamental stage, a real bridge between the safe environment of the hospital and the family cocoon. With meticulous preparation, sympathetic support and open communication, the neonatal nurse can ensure a calm and reassuring transition for parents and their child.

The role of the nurse
in post-neonatal monitoring

The transition from neonatology to home is a milestone in a newborn baby's health journey. While the role of the neonatal nurse is paramount during the hospital stay, his or her influence does not stop at the hospital gates. Post-neonatal monitoring is of vital importance, ensuring continuity of care and guaranteeing the safety and well-being of the infant.

Home visits :
   For some newborns, home visits may be organised, enabling the nurse to assess the child's environment, check that medical recommendations are being followed and provide support to parents.
Follow-up clinics :
   Many neonatal units offer post-neonatal clinics. The nurse plays a key role here, assessing the newborn's growth and development, administering vaccinations and making sure everything is going well.
Continuing education :
   As well as providing medical care, nurses also educate parents. Whether it's about nutrition, sleep, or the child's changing needs, the nurse provides advice and recommendations on how best to navigate this new stage.
Referral to other specialists:
   If the baby has specific needs, the nurse is often the first point of contact for referring parents to other professionals, such as physiotherapists, speech therapists or nutritionists.
Psychological support :
   The transition from hospital to home can be emotionally challenging for parents. The nurse is

there to listen, reassure and suggest appropriate resources if necessary.

Coordination with the paediatrician :

The nurse works closely with the newborn's paediatrician, ensuring that the medical follow-up is consistent and meets the child's specific needs.

Participation in research :

Many neonatal nurses take part in longitudinal studies, following the newborns they have cared for to understand the evolution of their health and contribute to the advancement of knowledge.

Post-neonatal monitoring by the nurse is essential to ensure holistic care for the newborn. Through their presence, expertise and dedication, nurses provide invaluable security for parents and play a decisive role in the child's health and development.

The transition to paediatric care

The world of neonatology is unique and specialised. But, like the metaphor of the bud turning into a flower, there comes a time when the newborn baby leaves this protective cocoon and is integrated into the continuum of paediatric care. This transition is essential to ensure continuity of care and to support families in this new phase of their child's life.

Initial assessment :

Once the baby is ready to be discharged from the neonatal unit, a comprehensive assessment is carried out to check the baby's state of health and identify any paediatric care needs.

Preparing parents :

The prospect of leaving the reassuring world of the neonatal unit can be frightening for many parents. The medical teams focus on education, preparing parents for what lies ahead, from regular appointments with the paediatrician to vaccinations and the child's development and growth.

Planning the transfer :

In collaboration with the paediatricians, a care plan is drawn up, ensuring that all relevant information is shared and that the next necessary appointments and follow-ups are scheduled.

Initial close monitoring :

In the first few weeks after discharge from the neonatal unit, babies are often closely monitored by the paediatrician to ensure that their transition goes smoothly and that they continue to grow and develop correctly.

Integration of specialists :

For certain children with specific needs, other specialists could be integrated into their follow-up, such as cardiologists, neurologists or speech therapists.

Emotional support :

As parents adjust to this new phase, it is crucial to offer them emotional support. Support groups, consultations with psychologists, or other resources can be offered to help them through this transition.

Continuing education :

A child's growth and development don't stop after neonatology. Parents continue to receive information on nutrition, sleep, developmental milestones and many other relevant topics as their child grows.

The transition to paediatric care is a fundamental stage in every child's medical journey. With the right support, open communication and careful planning, this transition can be made as smooth and seamless as possible for the child and their family.

Chapter 19:
NEURODEVELOPMENT
IN NEONATOLOGY

Foundations of neurodevelopment the premature baby

Premature birth poses a particular challenge in terms of neurological development. The brain of the premature baby is both vulnerable and plastic, which means that it is susceptible to being influenced, for good or ill, by its environment. To understand the subtleties of neurodevelopment in the premature baby, let's delve into this fascinating journey of growth and adaptation.

Embryonic stage: the basis of everything
Before birth, the foetal brain is already active, laying the foundations for what will become the child's neurological network. Neurons form, migrate and establish the first connections. This is a crucial period, and premature birth interrupts this process, moving it from the womb to the outside world.
Vulnerability of the premature brain :
Because of its incomplete maturation, the premature baby's brain is particularly vulnerable to aggression, whether physical, such as an injury, or chemical, such as an oxygen imbalance. These challenges can have consequences for cognitive, motor and sensory development.
Cerebral plasticity: a double-edged sword
Plasticity refers to the brain's ability to remodel itself in response to its environment. It is an astonishing ability, especially in premature

babies. It can enable remarkable recovery from injury, but it also means that negative experiences can have lasting consequences.

Targeted interventions :

Neonatal care seeks to minimise stress and encourage an environment conducive to brain development. This may involve methods such as skin-to-skin contact, controlled sensory stimulation or the use of music.

Longitudinal monitoring :

For premature babies, monitoring their neurological development does not stop when they leave hospital. Regular assessments enable us to detect any delays or deficits and intervene quickly.

The role of parents and carers :

Their role is essential in supporting the optimal neurological development of premature babies. Understanding, patience and commitment to appropriate interventions can make all the difference.

Research and hope :

Research into the neurodevelopment of premature babies is making great strides, offering hope for better interventions and even more positive results in the future.

The neurodevelopment of premature babies is a complex journey, fraught with pitfalls but also with resilience and potential. With medical advances, the in-depth understanding of healthcare professionals and the invaluable support of families, these little warriors have every chance of reaching their full potential.

Impact of care and environment on the developing brain

The development of a newborn baby's brain is a complex and dynamic process, particularly for babies born prematurely. Every experience, every stimulus, every deficiency can leave an imprint on this maturing brain. Understanding the impact of care and environment is crucial to optimising the neurological development of newborn babies.

The sensory environment :
Despite their vital role, neonatal units can be noisy and bright places. The brains of newborn babies, particularly premature babies, are sensitive to this sensory overload. A calm environment, subdued lighting and limited exposure to loud noises can promote healthy brain development.

Positive experiences :
Interventions such as skin-to-skin contact, parents' soothing voices and gentle touch help to strengthen neural connections. This positive stimulation can even reduce the effects of stressful experiences.

Stress and pain :
Medical procedures, even if necessary, can cause stress or pain to the newborn. Repeated exposure to stress can affect the way the brain deals with stress in the long term.

Nutrition :
The brain needs adequate nutrition to develop properly. An optimal intake of nutrients, particularly omega-3 fatty acids, is essential for the myelination of neurons and the formation of synapses.

Social interaction :

Babies' first interactions with their carers and parents play a decisive role in the development of their social and emotional skills. Constant emotional support, responses tailored to their needs and interactive stimulation are crucial.

Enriching the environment :

An environment rich in appropriate stimulation can accelerate brain development. This includes appropriate toys, music and even reading aloud.

Security and attachment :

A sense of security, reinforced by a strong attachment to parental figures, has a profoundly positive impact on brain development. It promotes emotional, cognitive and social growth.

The impact of drugs :

Certain drugs administered in neonatal care can have effects on the developing brain. It is therefore essential to closely monitor newborns on medication.

The importance of sleep :

Sleep plays a fundamental role in memory consolidation and brain maturation. Ensuring regular, undisturbed sleep cycles is therefore essential.

The first days, weeks and months of a baby's life are critical for its neurological development. Every intervention, every choice of environment, every interaction plays a part in shaping their neurological future. By understanding and respecting these nuances, carers and parents can provide the best possible foundation for the growth and development of these young lives.

Strategies to support optimal neural development

The brain of a newborn baby is an ever-evolving marvel, comparable to a blank canvas that gradually takes on new colours with each new experience. While the foundations of the brain are largely determined by genetics, it is the environment, early care and interaction that really shape it. Various strategies can be adopted to optimise neural development:

Appropriate sensory stimulation :
Exposing newborns to varied but not overloading stimuli, such as soft textures, soothing music or maternal smells, can strengthen neuronal connections.

Skin-to-skin contact :
This practice, also known as the 'kangaroo method', not only stimulates the production of oxytocin, the attachment hormone, but also promotes cognitive and emotional development.

Voice interaction :
Talking, singing or simply whispering to your baby stimulates their auditory development and strengthens their bond.

Optimum nutrition :
The right nutritional intake, rich in essential fatty acids, proteins and micronutrients, is crucial for brain development.

Stable environment :
A predictable and reassuring environment, where babies feel safe and comfortable, is conducive to calm neural development.

Visual stimulation :

Moving objects, contrasts and colours can help to develop a baby's vision, although excessive stimulation should be avoided.

Stress reduction :

A peaceful environment, reassuring routines and gentle medical interventions can help reduce levels of cortisol, the stress hormone, in newborn babies.

Games and exploration :

As babies grow, providing them with age-appropriate toys and encouraging them to explore their environment contributes to brain plasticity.

Reading :

Even if babies don't understand words, listening to stories and looking at pictures stimulates their imagination and curiosity.

Emotional bond :

Warm, loving and caring interactions not only strengthen the parent-child bond, but also stimulate the baby's emotional and social development.

Appropriate physical exercise :

Activities such as moving the baby's arms and legs, or "baby gymnastics" sessions, can strengthen coordination and motor development.

Cognitive stimulation :

Playing simple games, solving small problems and interacting with the environment helps to stimulate thinking and memory.

By combining tender care with appropriate stimulation, we can help sculpt baby's neural landscape, laying the foundations for a fulfilling cognitive, emotional and social future.

Chapter 20:
PALLIATIVE CARE IN NEONATOLOGY

When and why they are needed

Palliative care in neonatology involves the overall management of newborns with life-limiting illnesses or conditions incompatible with prolonged life. It is not just end-of-life care, but an approach that aims to improve the quality of life of the newborn and his or her family.

When necessary :

- **Serious congenital anomalies:** Some babies are born with anomalies that cannot be corrected surgically or that would result in great suffering or poor quality of life.
- **Severe neurological conditions:** Severe brain lesions, chromosomal abnormalities or metabolic diseases may limit the length and quality of life of the newborn.
- **Multi-system organ dysfunction:** For example, severe cardiac, renal or respiratory failure that does not respond to treatment.
- **Inevitable outcome:** In cases where death is imminent, whatever the interventions.

Why they are necessary :

- **Pain relief and comfort:** Palliative care ensures that the newborn receives the necessary medication and care to be as comfortable as possible, minimising pain and distress.
- **Emotional and psychological support:** They offer support to parents and families, helping them to navigate complex emotions and bereavement.

Informed decisions: They provide parents with comprehensive and understandable information to help them make informed decisions about their child's care.

Respect for the family's wishes: Palliative care takes account of the family's values, beliefs and wishes regarding their child's care.

Continuity of care: They offer continuity of care, ensuring that the needs of the newborn and their family are met at every stage, from diagnosis to outcome, including post-mortem support for the family.

Multidisciplinary approach: They involve a team of paediatricians, nurses, social workers, psychologists, spiritual therapists and other specialists to provide holistic care.

Neonatology, despite its advances, is faced with moments when recovery or prolonged survival is not possible. At these times, palliative care in neonatology offers a glimmer of humanity, ensuring that every newborn is treated with dignity, love and respect, and that every family is supported in their journey.

How to approach care end of life with compassion

Dealing with end-of-life care requires great sensitivity, empathy and understanding. For healthcare professionals, this is not only a clinical challenge, but also an emotional one, where the human approach comes first. Here's how it can be done with compassion:

Active listening: Being truly present and actively listening to the patient and their family allows us to understand their fears, needs and desires. It provides a space for them to express their feelings without judgement.

Open communication: It is essential to communicate clearly, honestly and sensitively. Information should be provided in an understandable way, while respecting the feelings and beliefs of the patient and family.

Presence and availability: Sometimes, the simple presence of a caring person can offer great comfort. Assuring the patient and their family that you are available to meet their needs or simply to be there with them is invaluable.

Emotional support: Recognising and validating the patient's and family's emotions. Offering psychological support or supportive therapy can be beneficial.

Respecting the patient's wishes: Everyone has their own wishes and beliefs regarding the end of life. It is essential to respect these choices, whether they be medical, spiritual or cultural.

Attention to detail: Little things, like creating a peaceful atmosphere in the room or playing the patient's favourite music, can make a big difference.

Spiritual support: For those for whom faith is important, providing spiritual support or facilitating access to religious services can be a source of comfort.

Continuity of care: Ensuring a smooth transition between hospital care and care at home, or between different providers, so that the patient always feels cared for and understood.

Family support: Families are also going through a difficult time. Offering support, education and resources can help them get through this period with strength and resilience.

Pain management: Ensure that the patient is as comfortable as possible by managing pain and other uncomfortable symptoms appropriately.

Personal reflection: As a healthcare professional, taking the time to reflect on your own feelings and beliefs around the end of life can help you to be more present and compassionate.

Approaching end-of-life care with compassion means looking beyond the illness and recognising the intrinsic value and dignity of each individual. It is at these poignant moments that the heart of the medical profession is revealed, where science meets humanity.

Support for families during these delicate moments

In the tumultuous world of neonatology, as medical teams focus on the vital care of infants, it is equally crucial to remember the families who navigate these uncharted waters. For many, these moments mark a complex mix of joy, anxiety, hope and uncertainty. Supporting these families during these delicate times is not just a kind gesture, it is an essential part of the healing and well-being process.

At the heart of this support is the recognition that every family is unique. Some seek to understand every medical detail, while others drown under the weight of information. Some find comfort in solitude, others in companionship. Listening thus becomes the most valuable tool. By actively listening, the medical team can identify the specific needs of each family and tailor support accordingly.

But listening is not enough. Families need to be reassured that their child is receiving the best possible care. They need to feel that they are an integral part of the care team. This means keeping them informed, involving them in medical decisions where possible, and respecting their choices and beliefs.

Educational resources also play a key role. By providing clear, understandable information about medical conditions, treatments and procedures, families feel more in control and better equipped to support their child.

However, emotional support remains essential. Families need spaces where they can express their fears, mourn their losses, celebrate the small victories and find hope in the darkest moments. This can be facilitated by psychological support teams, peer support groups or simply a member of the medical team willing to sit down and share a moment.

Supporting families at this delicate time is an act of humanity that recognises the complexity and depth of the human experience. It's a reassuring pat on the shoulder, a compassionate look, a listening ear, and above all, a heart open to the vulnerability of the other. In the ballet of neonatal care, it is this support that provides the silent but powerful music to which hope dances.

Chapter 21:
ENVIRONMENT AND LAYOUT
OF THE NEONATAL UNIT

The importance of a suitable environment: light, sound, temperature

Neonatology is much more than just a medical science; it is a delicate art of balancing cutting-edge technology with primordial human instinct. At the heart of this art lies the creation of an optimal environment for newborn babies, particularly those who are premature or require intensive care. The environment, influenced by factors such as light, sound and temperature, plays an essential role in the infant's development and well-being.

Take **light, for** example. In the womb, a foetus is protected from direct, bright light. In the neonatal unit, soft, subdued lighting mimics this environment, minimising excessive stimulation and encouraging regular sleep cycles, which are essential for cerebral and physical development. In addition, studies have shown that periods of darkness can help regulate the circadian rhythm of premature babies, promoting healthy sleep and better weight gain.

Sound is just as crucial. Neonatal units can be noisy, with constant alarms, conversations and machinery noise. An overly noisy environment can increase stress in newborns, affecting their heart rate, breathing and oxygenation levels. To minimise these effects, units are often designed to dampen noise, and staff are trained to speak softly. Soothing sounds, such as the mother's heartbeat or a gentle lullaby, can even be used to calm an agitated baby.

Finally, **temperature is of** vital importance. Newborn babies, especially premature ones, have not yet developed the ability to regulate their body temperature effectively. A controlled ambient temperature, combined with the use of heated blankets or incubators, helps to maintain a stable body temperature, which is essential for growth and metabolism.

Individually, each of these elements may seem small, but together they form a harmonious whole, a cocoon of care that supports every moment of a newborn baby's fragile life. In this carefully orchestrated environment, every detail counts, reflecting the delicacy and depth of the medical team's commitment to providing the best possible care. Ultimately, it is this meticulous attention to the environment that often makes the difference between survival and prosperity for these little creatures.

Design and layout :
of the traditional unit
to family units centred

The world of neonatology, once dominated by sterile visions of incubators in rows and monitors flashing, has undergone a radical transformation in recent decades. This evolution, driven by a better understanding of the emotional and physiological needs of newborns and their families, has redefined the very concept of the design and layout of neonatal care units.

Traditionally, neonatal units were clinical, functional and optimised spaces for nursing staff. Incubators were often grouped together in a large room, allowing care staff to monitor many babies at once. While this configuration was certainly efficient from an operational point of view, it often neglected the human aspect of care. Parents found themselves on the sidelines, only able to interact with their child for short periods and often separated by a pane of glass.

Awareness of the benefits of **family-centred units** has led to a redesign of neonatal units. These spaces are designed to put families at the heart of care, recognising their essential role as care partners for their children. In these units, parents have their own space, often equipped with a sofa or bed, allowing them to stay close to their baby day and night. This constant parental presence has been associated with better outcomes for newborn babies, including earlier discharge from hospital, better weight gain and greater emotional stability.

But the transition to centred family units is not just about adding space for parents. It's a transformation that takes into account natural light, soothing colours, natural materials and noise reduction. The result is an environment that not only supports the baby's well-being, but that of the whole family.

This transition from a purely clinical design to a family-centred space is not just a question of aesthetics or comfort. It's about recognising the importance of emotional ties in the healing process, accepting that parents are not just visitors but key players in their child's care, and adapting the environment accordingly.

These changes in the design and layout of neonatal units represent a move towards a more holistic approach to care, where the emotional and physical well-being of patients and their families is at the heart of every decision.

Impact on the well-being of newborns, families and staff

The design and structure of a neonatal unit are not simply a question of aesthetics or functionality; they have a profound effect on the well-being of everyone involved. Newborns, families and even medical staff all benefit from a well-designed unit.

For newborns: An optimised environment, focused on the child's well-being, promotes healthy development. Units that take account of natural light, minimise noise levels and offer spaces conducive to skin-to-skin contact between parent and child contribute to more stable growth and development in newborns. What's more, a serene, less stressful environment can have a positive influence on a baby's circadian rhythms, weight gain and even their ability to fight infection.

For families: Parenting a child in a neonatal unit can be a traumatic and stressful experience. Family-centred units recognise and value the role of the parent as a partner in care. They provide a space where parents can rest, recharge and spend quality time with their baby. This not only strengthens the bond between parent and child, but also gives parents a sense of involvement and control, reducing their stress and anxiety.

For staff: Nurses, doctors and other staff also benefit from a well-designed environment. Ergonomically designed workspaces improve efficiency, reduce fatigue and minimise errors. Spaces dedicated to relaxation and recuperation can help to manage the stress inherent in this type of work. What's more, by working in a unit that values collaboration between carers and families, staff often feel more satisfied and valued in their role, which can translate into better staff retention and improved quality of care.

Taking into account all aspects of well-being, for patients, their families and medical staff, is an investment that pays off. The impact is measured not only in terms of improved medical outcomes, but also in terms of satisfaction, strengthened relationships and a better overall experience for all.

Chapter 22:
INFECTION MANAGEMENT IN NEONATAL UNITS

Prevention, detection and treatment of common infections

In the delicate context of neonatal care, infection prevention is of vital importance. Newborn babies, particularly premature babies, have immature immune systems, making them particularly vulnerable to infection. Managing these infections requires an integrated approach involving prevention, early detection and appropriate treatment.

1. Prevention :

Hygiene measures: The first line of defence against infection is impeccable hygiene. This includes frequent and meticulous hand washing, and wearing sterile gloves, gowns and masks when handling newborns.

Isolation: Babies suspected or confirmed to be carrying an infection should be isolated to prevent spread.

Antibiotic prophylaxis: In certain cases, antibiotics can be administered as a preventive measure, particularly in high-risk babies.

Vaccinations: Some vaccinations can be given from birth, such as the hepatitis B vaccine.

2. Detection :

Continuous monitoring: Regular monitoring of vital signs can provide clues to possible infection.

Clinical signs: Irritability, lethargy, unstable body temperature, difficulty breathing or eating may be indicators of infection.

Laboratory tests: blood, urine or cerebrospinal samples are taken to detect the presence of bacteria or other pathogens.

3. Processing :

Antibiotic therapy: Once the infection has been confirmed, a targeted course of antibiotics is started. It is essential to choose the appropriate antibiotic depending on the infectious agent identified.

Support for vital functions: In severe cases, respiratory or cardiovascular assistance may be required.

Nutrition: Ensuring adequate nutrition is fundamental to supporting the baby's growth and helping to fight infection.

Parent education: Parents must be informed of the signs of infection and the measures to be taken at home, particularly with regard to hygiene and medication management.

Neonatology requires constant vigilance. Close collaboration between nursing staff and families is essential to prevent, detect and treat infections effectively, thereby guaranteeing the best chances of recovery for these fragile beings.

Hygiene protocols

Neonatology, with its highly vulnerable population, requires a highly specialised approach to hygiene. Hygiene protocols are rigorous and essential to prevent nosocomial infections, which can have serious or even fatal consequences for newborn babies.

1. Hand hygiene :

Frequency: Hands should be washed before and after each interaction with a newborn, after touching potentially contaminated surfaces, and before performing sterile procedures.

Technique: Hand washing should last at least 30 seconds using a mild soap and an appropriate technique to cover all surfaces. The use of hydroalcoholic solutions may be recommended in the absence of visible soiling.

2. Personal protective equipment (PPE) :

Sterile gloves: Worn for all invasive procedures or if in contact with secretions.

Gowns, masks and goggles: Used where there is a risk of spraying body secretions or during specific procedures.

3. Environmental hygiene :

Regular cleaning: Surfaces, floors, appliances and equipment must be cleaned and disinfected regularly using suitable products.

Waste management : Biomedical waste must be disposed of safely, according to strict protocols.

4. Hygiene of medical equipment :

Sterilisation: All equipment coming into direct contact with the newborn (probes, catheters) must be sterile.

Single use: Single-use devices should be discarded after a single use to avoid cross-contamination.

5. Isolation :

Cases of infection : Babies with a confirmed or suspected infection should be placed in isolation to prevent spread to other patients.

6. Training and awareness :

Nursing staff : Must be regularly trained and updated on hygiene protocols.

Families: They must be made aware of the importance of hygiene measures, particularly hand washing, when they are in contact with their child.

7. Monitoring and feedback :

   Epidemiological monitoring: Enables any epidemics or increases in infections to be detected quickly and protocols adapted accordingly.

   Feedback: Encourage staff to report any shortcomings or problems observed in the application of the protocols for continuous improvement.

Strict compliance with these neonatal hygiene protocols is vital to ensure the safety of the babies in our care. Everyone involved, from doctors to families, has a role to play in this chain of prevention.

Vaccination and prophylaxis in neonatology

Neonatology is a delicate area where newborn babies are cared for, many of whom are premature and have immature immune systems. This makes them particularly vulnerable to infection. Fortunately, medical science has developed ways of protecting these little patients through vaccination and prophylaxis.

1. Vaccination in neonatology :

   Importance: Even at this tender age, certain vaccinations are essential to protect newborn babies against potentially fatal diseases.

   BCG vaccine: Administered in some parts of the world to protect against tuberculosis.

   Hepatitis B vaccine: The first dose is often given shortly after birth, especially if the mother is a carrier of the hepatitis B virus.

   Passive vaccination: In some cases, newborns are given immunoglobulins, which are prefabricated antibodies, to provide temporary protection against certain diseases.

2. Prophylaxis in neonatology :

Antibiotic prophylaxis: In certain high-risk newborns, antibiotics can be administered from birth to prevent possible bacterial infection.

Antiviral prophylaxis: For newborns exposed to viruses such as HIV, antiviral drugs can be administered as prophylaxis.

Prophylaxis of haemolytic disease of the newborn: Rh-negative mothers who give birth to an Rh-positive baby can receive an injection of anti-D immunoglobulin to prevent this condition in subsequent pregnancies.

Prophylaxis of retinopathy of prematurity: In some cases, rigorously controlled oxygen therapy is used to prevent this eye disease in premature babies.

3. Specific considerations :

Consent: Parents must be informed of all the benefits, risks and alternatives before administering a vaccine or prophylactic treatment.

Monitoring: After vaccination or prophylaxis, it is essential to monitor newborns for possible side effects or reactions.

Planning: An appropriate vaccination schedule must be drawn up to ensure that the newborn receives all the necessary doses of each vaccine.

Vaccination and prophylaxis play a crucial role in neonatology, providing a line of defence against diseases that could otherwise have devastating consequences for these young patients. The key is careful implementation, transparent communication with parents and careful monitoring to ensure the safety and well-being of the newborn.

Chapter 23:
ATYPICAL CAREER PATHS :
GEMINI, MALFORMATIONS, ETC.

Managing complex and rare situations

Neonatology, although focused on the care of newborn babies, encompasses a wide range of medical conditions, from the most common to the rarest. These complex situations require not only cutting-edge medical expertise, but also finesse in communication and an empathetic understanding of the families affected.

1. Recognition and diagnosis :
    Careful monitoring: When faced with atypical symptoms, constant monitoring of the newborn is essential to detect the early signs of a rare condition.
    Differential diagnosis: Using a methodical approach to eliminate common causes and direct investigations towards rarer conditions.
    Cutting-edge technologies: The use of genetic and molecular diagnostics can help identify rare conditions.
2. Intervention and management :
    Individualised treatment plan: Each rare condition may require a unique approach, combining standard therapies with experimental or innovative treatments.
    Specialist consultation: Calling on experts in specific fields, sometimes even internationally, may be necessary for advice or treatment recommendations.
    Adaptability: Established protocols may not exist for certain rare conditions, requiring flexibility and creativity in management.

3. Emotional and psychological support :

   Communication with families: Explain the complex nature of the condition and possible uncertainties with empathy, and provide clear, honest information.

   Psychological support: Offer parents meetings with psychologists or social workers to help them deal with stress and emotions.

   Support networks: Direct families to associations or support groups specialising in rare conditions to share experiences and get advice.

4. Interprofessional collaboration :

   Multidisciplinary team: The management of rare conditions may require the expertise of many specialists, from genetics to surgery.

   Research and training: Collaboration with research centres and academic institutions can provide valuable insights and contribute to the ongoing training of the care team.

5. Anticipation and planning :

   Long-term plan: Anticipate the newborn's future needs as he or she grows, particularly in terms of medical monitoring, development and educational support.

   Transition to specialist paediatric care: Ensuring a smooth transition from the neonatal department to other specialties that will care for the child as he or she grows.

Complex and rare situations in neonatology test the skills and resilience of the medical team. They require a combination of knowledge, clinical skills, compassion and collaboration to provide the best possible care for newborns and support their families through unexpected challenges.

Care coordination
for multiple situations

In neonatology, it is not uncommon to encounter newborns with several simultaneous complications, requiring multidisciplinary care. Ensuring effective coordination of care in these situations is essential to optimising the newborn's well-being and supporting his or her family.

1. Initial assessment :
As soon as the baby is born, a thorough assessment is carried out. This assessment must be comprehensive and enable the various conditions or anomalies that may affect the baby to be identified. Tests and examinations, from the simplest to the most sophisticated, are used to establish a precise diagnosis.

2. Drawing up a care plan :
Once all the conditions have been identified, a care plan is drawn up. This plan must take into account the severity of each condition, how they may interact with each other and treatment priorities.

3. Involvement of specialists :
Depending on the complications diagnosed, different specialists may be involved:
- Cardiologists for heart problems,
- Neurologists for neurological complications,
- Orthopaedists for musculoskeletal disorders,
- And many more.

4. Interdisciplinary communication :
Regular meetings between healthcare professionals are essential. These exchanges help to ensure consistent care, monitor the baby's progress, adjust treatments and coordinate care.

5. Support for parents :
Parents often find themselves at a loss when faced with the complexities of caring for their child. They need to be informed, supported and involved in decisions. Regular

meetings with the medical team, psychologists and social workers can help them navigate through this difficult period.

6. Ongoing monitoring :
Regular follow-up is essential to monitor the progress of the various conditions, the effectiveness of treatments and to detect any new complications. The baby's medical file must be kept up to date and accessible to all the professionals involved.

7. Planning the outing :
When it is time to leave the neonatal unit, a comprehensive discharge plan is drawn up. This plan must include all information relating to home care, medication, future medical appointments and available support measures.

Coordinating care in neonatology is a complex process, but one that is essential to ensure the well-being of newborn babies in multiple situations. Every healthcare professional has a key role to play, and collaboration, communication and commitment are at the heart of this process.

Case studies and feedback

Dive into the real world of neonatology through case studies and feedback. These true stories, drawn from clinical reality, offer a unique perspective on the challenges, successes and lessons learned in caring for newborn babies. They reflect not only medical science, but also the humanity and compassion that surround this specialised field.

1. The case of Léo :
Léo was born at 25 weeks' gestation, weighing just over half a kilo. His first days were marked by respiratory distress requiring intubation. Over the weeks, with the

constant attention of the neonatology team, Léo progressed, despite ups and downs.

Feedback: Perseverance, patience and collaboration between professionals and the family are crucial to overcoming the challenges of very premature babies.

2. The case of Aisha :

Aisha, born at full term, developed severe jaundice on the third day after birth. Proactive monitoring revealed Rh incompatibility, which was treated with intense phototherapy.

Feedback: All newborns, even those born at term, can have complications. Careful monitoring is essential.

3. The case of Miguel :

Miguel was born with a complex heart defect. From birth, he was cared for by a multidisciplinary team, including cardiologists, surgeons and specialist nurses.

Feedback: Congenital anomalies can be unpredictable, but with the right preparation and coordination, many children like Miguel can lead a normal life.

4. Nora's case :

Nora, who was born prematurely, contracted a nosocomial infection in the neonatal unit. This led to weeks of antibiotics and intensive care.

Case study: Hygiene protocols are vital. An infection can radically change a newborn's care.

Each case in neonatology is unique, but they all offer valuable lessons. These case studies illustrate the need for ongoing training, close collaboration between professionals, and transparent communication with families. Behind each story lies not only science and technology, but also a profound humanity. These experiences serve as a reminder of the importance of the role of neonatal carers and the profound impact of their interventions.

Chapter 24:
REHABILITATION AND PHYSIOTHERAPY IN NEONATOLOGY

Importance of early mobilisation

Early mobilisation is the process of stimulating and encouraging movement and physical activity in newborn babies as soon as possible after birth, particularly those who are hospitalised or have special needs. This practice, although relatively new to neonatology, has gained ground thanks to numerous studies showing its potential benefits.

1. Neurological development :
The first days and weeks of a newborn's life are crucial for brain development. Early mobilisation can play a role in stimulating the brain, facilitating the myelination of neurons and promoting neuroplasticity. This can have long-term implications for the child's cognitive and motor development.

2. Muscle and bone function :
Early mobilisation helps to strengthen muscles and improve bone density. For premature babies, who often spend long periods in bed, this can prevent muscle atrophy and promote healthy bone growth.

3. Sensory stimulation :
Movement encourages interaction with the environment, providing tactile, visual and auditory stimulation. These multisensory experiences are essential for neurosensory development.

4. Improved cardiorespiratory function :
Active movement and positioning can help improve circulation, oxygenation and lung function, reducing the risk of complications associated with immobility.

5. Emotional and social well-being :
Physical interactions, such as skin-to-skin contact with parents during mobilisation, strengthen the bond of attachment and provide emotional comfort for the newborn.

6. Preparing for the trip :
A baby who has been actively mobilised is often more alert, has improved muscle tone and may be better prepared for the transition home.

7. Reducing complications :
Early mobilisation can reduce the risk of complications such as developmental delay, muscular atrophy and respiratory problems, particularly in premature babies.

Early mobilisation in neonatology is a patient-centred approach that recognises the potential of every newborn to grow and develop, even in adverse medical circumstances. It requires a dedicated team, appropriate resources and specific training. However, with good practice and increased awareness, it can transform the developmental journey of many newborns, offering a better quality of life and a brighter future.

Techniques and routine operations

Neonatology, a medical speciality dedicated to the care of newborn babies, particularly premature babies and babies with special medical needs, involves a wide range of techniques and procedures. Here is an overview of the most common techniques and procedures:

Endotracheal intubation: This procedure involves inserting a tube into the baby's trachea to ensure a safe passage of air, generally as part of respiratory assistance.

Mechanical ventilation: Used for babies who have difficulty breathing on their own, this machine pushes air into the lungs through the endotracheal tube.

Surfactant : Often given to premature babies to treat or prevent respiratory distress syndrome. Surfactant is a natural substance that reduces the tension inside the pulmonary alveoli.

Phototherapy: A method used to treat neonatal jaundice. The baby is placed under a special light that helps break down bilirubin, a substance that can build up in the baby's blood.

Central venous catheterisation: involves inserting a catheter into a large vein, usually to administer medication or nutrients.

Enteral feeding: The administration of nutrients directly into the stomach or intestine, either through a nasal tube or a gastric tube.

Parenteral nutrition: Provides nutrients directly into the bloodstream, often used when enteral nutrition is not possible or insufficient.

Cerebral ultrasound: An imaging tool used to assess the brain of premature babies, looking for signs of haemorrhage or other abnormalities.

Cardiac monitoring: Uses electrodes to monitor the baby's heart rate and rhythm.

Pulse oximetry: A non-invasive method of monitoring oxygen levels in the blood.

Echocardiography: An ultrasound scan of the heart to visualise its structure and function.

Metabolic tests: Carried out to detect rare but serious metabolic or genetic diseases.

Culture and sensitivity tests: Used to diagnose and treat infections.

Abdominal ultrasound: An imaging tool for visualising the internal organs of the abdomen, often used to diagnose or monitor conditions such as bowel perforation.

145

These interventions, among many others, enable healthcare professionals to monitor, diagnose and treat a variety of medical conditions in newborns, ensuring that they receive the best possible care during this critical period of their lives.

Working with specialists rehabilitation

Collaboration with neonatal rehabilitation specialists is essential to ensure comprehensive care for newborn babies. These specialists play a vital role in guiding infants and their families through the various stages of recovery and development.

Babies in the neonatal unit, particularly those who are premature or have special medical needs, may present developmental challenges or delays in crucial stages of their growth. This is where physiotherapists, occupational therapists, speech therapists and other specialists come in. They provide their expertise to stimulate the motor development, coordination, communication and sensory skills of infants.

Working closely with these experts enables the neonatal team to offer targeted interventions. For example, a physiotherapist could help an infant strengthen his muscles and develop his movements, while a speech therapist would work on skills such as sucking, swallowing and, later, vocal skills.

Rehabilitation specialists can also provide valuable advice to parents, helping them to understand their baby's unique needs and put in place strategies to support their baby's development at home. This parental education is fundamental, as it lays a solid foundation for the continued growth and well-being of the newborn.

The collaboration doesn't stop when the child leaves the neonatal unit. Often, these specialists continue to follow the child as he or she grows, ensuring that all stages of development are reached and providing interventions as required.

Collaboration with rehabilitation specialists enriches the neonatal experience, offering holistic care that goes beyond immediate medical care to embrace every aspect of the infant's well-being and development. This integrated approach ensures that every baby has the best possible chance to thrive and reach his or her full potential.

Chapter 25:
GENETICS AND NEONATOLOGY

Introduction to genetics
in neonatology

Genetics in neonatology opens a fascinating window onto the complex world of biological inheritance and its influence on the health of newborn babies. This intersection between genetics and neonatal medicine offers valuable insights into understanding, diagnosing and, in some cases, treating conditions that affect infants from birth.

1. The basis of genetics:
Every human being has a unique set of genetic information, or DNA, that determines everything from eye colour to predisposition to disease. This information is contained in genes, which are organised into structures called chromosomes.

2. Genetics and conception:
At conception, the embryo receives half of its genes from each parent, giving rise to a unique set of genetic information. It is this process that determines the individual's hereditary characteristics.

3. Genetic anomalies in neonatology:
Certain genetic abnormalities can lead to congenital malformations or hereditary diseases. Sometimes these conditions are identified before birth through prenatal tests. Other times, they are only discovered after birth, when an infant presents specific symptoms.

4. Genetic testing in neonatology:
There are a variety of genetic tests available for newborn babies. Newborn screening, for example, is a common procedure that tests infants for a range of genetic, metabolic and endocrine conditions.

5. The impact of genetics on treatment:
Understanding the genetics of a condition can have major implications for treatment. In some cases, it may even lead to specific therapeutic interventions or recommendations for supportive care.

6. The future of genetics in neonatology:
With advances in technology and research, the field of neonatal genetics continues to evolve at a rapid pace. New discoveries could offer even more targeted solutions for newborns with genetic anomalies or diseases.

Neonatal genetics is a rapidly expanding field that promises to improve the understanding, diagnosis and treatment of conditions that affect newborn babies. By offering insights into each individual's unique genetic code, it paves the way for personalised medicine that can be tailored to the specific needs of each infant.

Implications for diagnosis and care

Advances in neonatal genetics have transformed the way we approach the diagnosis and care of newborn babies. By delving into the very heart of the genetic code, we can now predict, diagnose and, in many cases, effectively treat conditions that were once poorly understood or went unnoticed.

From the very first moments of life, a baby's genetic make-up can reveal vital clues about its state of health. Thanks to modern diagnostic tools, rare or potentially dangerous conditions can be identified quickly, enabling early intervention. This is crucial because, for many neonatal conditions, the speed of intervention is crucial to the prognosis.

Beyond simple diagnosis, genetic knowledge also influences care. For example, pharmacogenomics, a branch of genetics that studies the interaction between genes and drugs, can help determine the most appropriate dose or type of drug for a newborn baby, based on its genetic profile. This makes it possible to avoid potentially harmful side effects and optimise the effectiveness of treatments.

Genetics in neonatology also has major implications for families. When a genetic condition is identified in a newborn, this can lead to testing of family members, sometimes revealing genetic risks of which they were unaware. In addition, by having a better understanding of the genetics of a condition, healthcare professionals can offer more informed support and advice to parents, helping them to navigate the complex and emotional challenges of caring for their child.

Finally, genetics is pushing back the boundaries of what is possible in neonatal care. With the emergence of innovative gene therapies, we are approaching a time when previously incurable diseases could be treated, or even cured, by directly targeting the defective genes.

The implications of neonatal genetics for diagnosis and care are profound. It offers exciting avenues for personalised medicine, improving prospects for many newborns and illuminating the path to their care, while supporting their families along the way.

Genetic counselling and family support

Genetic counselling in neonatology has established itself as a central element of holistic family care. By combining science, empathy and education, it aims to guide families through the complexities of genetics while supporting them emotionally.

When a newborn is found to have a genetic abnormality or hereditary disease, the emotions can be overwhelming for parents. They often ask questions like: "Why is this happening to us?", "What does this mean for my child's future?" or "Is there a risk for future children? This is where genetic counselling comes in, offering clear, factual answers to these questions.

The genetic counsellor, a specialist trained to interpret genetic information and translate it into understandable terms, assists parents in their quest for understanding. They provide detailed information on the nature of the anomaly or disease, the implications for the child and the family, and the treatment and care options available.

But as well as providing information, the genetic counsellor plays an essential role in providing emotional support. Faced with often unexpected news, parents can feel a mixture of shock, sadness, anger and confusion. The counsellor provides a safe space where parents can express their emotions, ask questions and find comfort.

Genetic counselling does not stop at the neonatal period. As the child grows, questions may arise about aspects such as schooling, reproduction or even social life. The counsellor remains a valuable ally, guiding the family every step of the way.

In addition, the genetic counsellor can also help assess the risks for other family members, particularly siblings or future children. By providing information on the genetic tests available and advising on procreation decisions, he or she supports the family as a whole.

Genetic counselling in neonatology is more than just passing on information. It is a true partnership between the counsellor and the family, aimed at providing both knowledge and emotional support. In the complex and sometimes confusing maze of genetics, the counsellor acts as a guide, anchor and confidant, ensuring that each family feels enlightened, supported and understood.

Chapter 26:
THE IMPORTANCE OF SKIN-TO-SKIN CONTACT AND HUMAN CONTACT

Proven benefits
skin-to-skin contact

Skin-to-skin contact, often referred to as the "kangaroo method", is a practice that encourages mothers or fathers to place their newborns on their bare chests, thereby promoting direct skin-to-skin contact. This seemingly simple technique has profound and scientifically proven benefits for the newborn, the mother and the parent-child relationship. Here's a fluid exploration of these benefits:

From the very first moments of life, skin-to-skin contact establishes a secure environment for the newborn. In the reassuring warmth of their parents' skin, babies find a space that reminds them of their mother's womb. This gentle transition from the intrauterine world to the outside environment stabilises the baby's heart and breathing rhythms. He feels less stress, which translates into less frequent crying and palpable relaxation.

Direct skin contact also helps to regulate the temperature of the newborn. The mother's temperature naturally adjusts to meet her baby's needs, warming or cooling as required. This is particularly beneficial for premature babies, who often have difficulty maintaining their own body temperature.

On a physiological level, skin-to-skin contact also encourages the colonisation of the baby's skin by the mother's beneficial bacteria, contributing to the formation of a healthy skin microbiome, an essential first step in the establishment of a robust immune system.

But the benefits of skin-to-skin contact go beyond simple physiology. For the mother, this intimacy boosts the release of oxytocin, often called the "love hormone". It promotes maternal attachment, helps reduce post-partum stress and even stimulates lactation, making breast-feeding easier.

The kangaroo method has also shown benefits for the development of a baby's brain. Children who have benefited from regular skin-to-skin contact tend to have a better response to stress, improved social skills and even better long-term cognition.

And the benefits are not limited to mother and child. Fathers who practise skin-to-skin contact with their newborns also develop a deeper attachment and feel more involved and competent in their parental roles.

Skin-to-skin contact is much more than just an embrace. It's a delicate dance of physiology and emotion, weaving a strong bond between parent and child, laying the foundations for a healthy, loving relationship for years to come.

Practical implementation and safety instructions

The implementation of skin-to-skin contact, although simple in theory, requires certain precautions and guidelines to guarantee the safety of the newborn and the parent. The integration of this practice into neonatal care must be carried out with rigour and care. Here is a fluid presentation of the practical implementation and safety instructions:

Practical implementation :

Preparation: Make sure the room is at a comfortable temperature to avoid any risk of hypothermia for the baby. The environment should be calm, with subdued lighting if possible.

Position: Whether mother or father, the person should be in a semi-recumbent position, with back support. Use cushions or pillows for extra comfort.

Dressing the baby: Newborns should be undressed right down to their nappy and, if possible, covered with a cap to keep their head warm.

Placement: Gently place the baby on the parent's chest, with the head turned to the side to ensure easy breathing. The baby's head should be level with the chest, making it easy to listen to the parent's heartbeat.

Blanket: Use a blanket or light sheet to cover baby's back, keeping him warm.

Duration: Ideally, skin-to-skin contact should last at least an hour or more, as this gives enough time to go through several cycles of sleep and wakefulness.

Safety instructions :

Supervision: It is essential that the parent is fully conscious and alert during the session, avoiding sedative drugs or excessive fatigue.

No sleep: To avoid any risk of falling or suffocating, the parent should not fall asleep with the baby on top of him or her. If the parent feels that he or she is about to fall asleep, it is best to put the baby back in the cot.

Breathing: Always make sure that your baby's nose and mouth are not blocked and that he can breathe freely.

Smokers: Parents who smoke should avoid skin-to-skin contact immediately after smoking, as tobacco residue can be harmful to the baby.

Baby's health: If the newborn has any particular health problems, it is essential to consult a health professional before starting practice.

Hygiene: Before starting the session, parents should wash their hands thoroughly.

Skin-to-skin contact is a powerful intervention which, when implemented correctly, can offer a myriad of benefits for both newborn and parent. However, safety must always come first.

Chapter 27:
NEONATAL EYE CARE

Understanding retinopathy of prematurity

As far as intrauterine maturation is concerned, each organ develops at its own pace. The eye, that delicate organ that opens us up to the outside world, is no exception to the rule. However, when a baby enters the world prematurely, this development is interrupted, and the eye may not be completely ready to face its new environment. This is where retinopathy of prematurity (ROP) comes in.

ROP is a condition that mainly affects the blood vessels of the retina, the thin membrane at the back of the eye that captures light and allows us to see. In premature babies, the vascularisation of the retina is not always complete. Once outside the womb, factors such as fluctuating oxygen levels can trigger abnormal growth of blood vessels. These new vessels are fragile and can bleed, leading to a risk of retinal detachment and, potentially, blindness.

It is fascinating to remember that this condition was almost unknown before the advent of modern care for premature babies. It is a paradoxical consequence of the success of modern medicine: by saving lives younger than ever before, we have faced challenges that nature had never foreseen.

Understanding and managing POR requires close collaboration between neonatologists and ophthalmologists. Regular retinal examinations of at-risk babies are crucial, and treatments such as laser therapy or cryotherapy may be necessary to prevent complications.

But beyond science and medicine, POR reminds us that every stage of foetal development is a miracle of balance, and that life, even at its earliest stages, is both robust and vulnerable. It reminds us of the importance of vigilance and prevention, but also of hope in the face of medical challenges.

Monitoring and treatment

The monitoring and treatment of retinopathy of prematurity (ROP) form an essential duo in the management of this condition, ensuring that our smallest patients have the best possible chance of preserving their sight. Let's find out how, in a meticulous medical choreography, specialists tackle this complication.

When the sun begins to break through, the birds sing, signalling the start of a new dawn. In the same way, the first moments of a premature baby's life are punctuated by signals, measurements and surveillance. POR, with its potentially serious implications for eyesight, is the focus of particular attention.

Monitoring: It all starts with identifying babies at risk. Generally speaking, it is the most premature babies, often born before 32 weeks' gestation or weighing less than 1,500 grams at birth, who are most likely to develop POR. These babies will be closely monitored by specialist paediatric ophthalmologists. Using an ophthalmoscope, the ophthalmologist examines the baby's retina for signs of abnormal vascularisation. These examinations generally begin 4 to 6 weeks after birth and continue until the retina is completely vascularised or the disease is treated.

Treatment: If POR progresses to a stage requiring treatment, several options are available. Laser therapy is the most commonly used. It aims to stop the growth of abnormal blood vessels by 'burning' the peripheral areas of the retina that are not properly vascularised. Another method is cryotherapy, which uses cold to achieve the same objective. In some cases, drug injections or even surgery may be necessary.

The choice of treatment depends on the stage of the disease, its location in the eye and the preferences of the specialist. One thing is constant, however: the need for prompt intervention. Acting early is crucial to preventing the long-term complications of POR, such as retinal detachment or blindness.

Beyond the tools and techniques, the management of POR is a testament to the dedication of the medical teams. It is the silent promise made to each premature baby: "We are watching over you, every beat of your heart, every breath, every ray of light that enters your eyes. We're here, and we'll do everything we can to give you the best possible start in life."

Prevention and awareness

In the delicate and nuanced world of neonatology, prevention and awareness play a central role. They are the pillars of safeguarding fragile and promising lives. Like a gentle melody guiding the steps of a dance, prevention lights the way, while awareness-raising forges links of understanding and empathy between healthcare professionals, parents and society. Let's dive into a world where every gesture, every word and every action counts.

From the very first moments of life, prevention is an integral part of neonatal care. Every measure, every protocol and every recommendation is designed to reduce risks and guarantee the well-being of newborn babies. Professionals' hands are carefully washed, care areas are meticulously disinfected, and equipment is scrupulously checked. Everything is orchestrated to prevent complications, whether nosocomial infections, trauma or medical errors.

But prevention goes well beyond the walls of neonatal units. It often begins well before birth, with prenatal advice to future parents on subjects such as nutrition, stopping smoking, limiting alcohol consumption and avoiding potentially harmful drugs. The aim of this advice is to avoid premature birth and ensure a healthy pregnancy.

Awareness-raising plays an equally vital role. Healthcare professionals make parents aware of their newborn's specific needs, educating them about the care to be given, the importance of skin-to-skin contact, and the signals to look out for. Raising awareness also helps to break down the stigma associated with prematurity or specific medical conditions, promoting understanding and acceptance.

At a societal level, awareness-raising aims to inform the general public about the challenges associated with neonatology, encourage support and promote research. It is a reminder of the importance of solidarity and community support for families navigating the world of neonatology.

In this way, prevention and awareness go hand in hand, forming an unbreakable alliance in the service of the most vulnerable. In this dance of life, they remind us that every moment is precious and that, together, we can make a difference.

Chapter 28:
CARDIAC CARE IN NEONATOLOGY

Congenital heart defects: detection and management

In the vast world of neonatology, the existence of congenital heart defects (CHDs) remains one of the major concerns of healthcare professionals. These anomalies, which affect the heart of the newborn from the moment of conception, are both complex to detect and to manage, requiring specialised expertise and seamless coordination of care. Understanding these anomalies means delving into the mysteries of the human heart.

The heart, such a vital organ, beats from the very first moments of conception, propelling life with every beat. But sometimes abnormalities occur in its formation, giving rise to CCAs. These deviations can be minor or critical, but all require special attention.

Early detection of ACC is essential. In many cases, the first signs can be identified during prenatal ultrasound scans. Thanks to modern technology, foetal cardiologists are able to obtain a detailed image of the foetal heart, making it possible to identify anomalies such as ventricular septal defects, tetralogies of Fallot or coarctations of the aorta. When an abnormality is suspected, more detailed examinations, such as foetal echocardiography, can be carried out.

At birth, clinical signs can also indicate the presence of CCA. Cyanosis (a bluish tinge to the skin), respiratory distress or poor weight gain may alert medical staff. Tests such as postnatal echocardiography or electrocardiograms can confirm the diagnosis.

Managing CCAs is just as delicate as detecting them. It requires a multidisciplinary approach, involving paediatric cardiologists, cardiac surgeons, specialist nurses and, of course, parents. Depending on the severity of the anomaly, different interventions may be considered: medication, cardiac catheterisation or open-heart surgery. Each decision is taken by carefully weighing up the risks and benefits for the newborn.

In this journey through the ACC, support for families is fundamental. The diagnosis of a cardiac anomaly in a newborn baby can be devastating for parents. Healthcare professionals have a crucial role to play in providing education, support and guidance, ensuring that every family feels supported and informed at every stage.

Ultimately, ACCs are a reminder of the fragility, but also the resilience, of life. Thanks to medical advances, many children born with these anomalies can now lead full and rich lives, bearing witness to the strength of the human heart and the determination of the medical teams working alongside them.

Collaboration with paediatric cardiologists

At the heart of the complex world of neonatology, collaboration with paediatric cardiologists is an essential step in ensuring optimal care for newborns with congenital heart defects or other cardiac problems. This professional alliance, based on the exchange of skills and transparent communication, plays a vital role in saving lives and ensuring a healthy future for the smallest among us.

The first few days of a newborn's life are crucial, and when a heart problem is detected, every second counts. This is where the paediatric cardiologist, a specialist in children's hearts, comes in, offering his expertise to decipher the mysteries of the young heart. In a neonatal unit, his presence is synonymous with hope, rapid intervention and appropriate strategies.

As soon as an abnormality is suspected, whether as a result of clinical symptoms, routine tests or a prenatal ultrasound scan, the paediatric cardiologist is called in. His role? To confirm the diagnosis, assess the seriousness of the condition and define the action plan. This may include medication, non-surgical procedures such as catheterisation, or more extensive surgery.

But beyond these medical skills, this specialist plays an essential role as a bridge between neonatology and cardiology. Working hand in hand with neonatologists, they ensure that the care provided is perfectly adapted to the specific cardiac needs of each infant. This collaboration also extends to continuing education: the paediatric cardiologist can offer information and training sessions to neonatology teams, ensuring that knowledge is constantly updated.

The relationship doesn't stop there. Parents, who are often anxious and overwhelmed by uncertainty, benefit greatly from this collaboration. Thanks to their in-depth knowledge of paediatric cardiac pathologies, paediatric cardiologists are able to explain the situation clearly, offer perspectives and guide parents through their child's medical journey.

Collaboration between neonatologists and paediatric cardiologists is much more than just professional coexistence. It is the guarantee of a holistic and integrated approach to care, where each area of expertise is put to work for the well-being of the newborn. In this medical ballet, each player, aware of the importance of his or her role, strives to do his or her best to offer a radiant future to these little beating hearts.

Case studies and research

Neonatology is a rich and complex field in which theory and practice are closely intertwined. Case studies offer healthcare professionals a unique opportunity to learn, adapt and constantly improve their methods. By immersing themselves in real-life situations, they are able to better grasp the dynamics of care, the challenges encountered and the solutions implemented.

Imagine Lisa, a premature baby born at 28 weeks, showing signs of respiratory distress from the very first moments of her life. The heart monitors also show irregularities. The neonatal team was immediately alerted and called in the paediatric cardiologist for an assessment. An echocardiogram was performed, revealing an interventricular communication (IVC), a congenital heart condition common in premature babies.

This case highlights the need for rapid and coordinated intervention. Initial management includes the administration of medication to support cardiac function and ventilation to help Lisa breathe. The paediatric cardiologist, in close collaboration with the neonatologist, decides on the best approach: monitoring the evolution of the IVC in the hope of spontaneous closure, or considering surgical intervention if necessary.

Another example would be Maxime, a full-term newborn who developed severe jaundice in the first 48 hours of life. Despite phototherapy, his bilirubin levels continued to rise, raising concerns about a possible Crigler-Najjar syndrome, a rare genetic condition affecting bilirubin metabolism. The team is calling in a geneticist to confirm the diagnosis, determine the type of syndrome and guide treatment.

This case study would highlight the importance of early detection, rapid intervention and interdisciplinary collaboration in managing rare but potentially life-threatening conditions.

Each neonatal case report is a window onto a multitude of clinical situations. They provide invaluable learning opportunities, enabling professionals to understand the nuances of neonatal care, hone their skills and ensure optimal management of newborns. Building on these studies, the world of neonatology continues to evolve, ensuring ever safer and more effective care for the most vulnerable.

Chapter 29:
NEONATOLOGY
AND THE ENVIRONMENT

Impact of pollutants and toxins on newborn babies

In a constantly changing world, the pollutants and toxins present in our environment are giving rise to growing concern, particularly as regards their impact on the most vulnerable: newborn babies. These substances, whether present in the air we breathe, the water we drink or in our food, can have serious consequences for the development and health of infants.

From the beginning of intrauterine life, the foetus is exposed to the maternal environment. Toxins can cross the placenta, creating a potential risk for foetal development. For example, smoking during pregnancy exposes the foetus to nicotine and other harmful compounds, increasing the risk of premature birth, low birth weight and respiratory problems.

Heavy metals, such as lead and mercury, can also seriously affect the neurological development of newborn babies. Early exposure to lead, even at low levels, is associated with learning disabilities and reduced IQ. Mercury, often found in certain types of fish, can disrupt the development of the brain and nervous system.

Endocrine disruptors, such as bisphenols and certain phthalates, found in many plastics and household products, are another major concern. These compounds can mimic or interfere with the body's natural hormones, disrupting the endocrine and reproductive systems.

Postnatal exposure, particularly through breastfeeding, can also be a source of concern. Although breast milk is ideally suited to the nutritional needs of the newborn and offers many immune benefits, it can also be a vector for the transmission of certain toxins accumulated in the mother's body.

The air that newborn babies breathe is another source of exposure. Air pollutants such as fine particles and volatile organic compounds can aggravate or trigger respiratory conditions such as asthma.

In the face of these challenges, a proactive approach is essential. Global initiatives to reduce pollution, combined with individual measures such as a balanced diet, avoiding smoking or limiting exposure to certain chemical substances, can help protect the health of newborn babies.

Science is still studying the precise impact of pollutants on neonatal health, but one thing is clear: prevention and awareness-raising are crucial steps in ensuring a healthy future for our children.

Green initiatives in neonatal units

Growing awareness of environmental impacts has led to an ecological revolution in various sectors, including the medical field. Neonatology units, aware of their crucial role in the first days of a newborn baby's life and the large volume of medical waste they can generate, have not been left behind. They have undertaken numerous initiatives to reduce their carbon footprint while guaranteeing high-quality care.

The first step for many units was to carry out an ecological audit to identify areas for improvement. This often revealed that most waste came from single-use products, such as nappies, gloves, syringes and other medical consumables.

Given this situation, a number of solutions were considered:

Reuse and sterilisation: Rather than systematically throwing away after a single use, some units have invested in sterilisable and reusable equipment. Although this may require an initial investment, it considerably reduces waste in the long term.

Eco-responsible purchasing: Buying eco-designed products or products made from recycled materials, and choosing suppliers with sustainable practices, also helps to reduce our ecological footprint.

Waste management: Selective waste management means that hazardous waste is recycled as much as possible and treated appropriately.

Energy savings: Switching to LED lighting, optimising heating and cooling systems, and using energy-efficient appliances all significantly reduce electricity consumption.

Training and awareness-raising: Staff are trained in best ecological practices, and awareness-raising campaigns can also be run for parents.

Green features: Introducing plants or vertical gardens can not only improve air quality, but also provide a more soothing, natural environment.

Community initiatives: In addition to internal practices, some units organise reforestation campaigns, local clean-ups or support ecological projects in their community.

These initiatives show that it is entirely possible to reconcile cutting-edge medical care with respect for the environment. With the will and commitment, neonatology units can play a leading role in the transition to more sustainable healthcare.

Awareness-raising and education

Awareness and education are two fundamental pillars in ensuring the success of any medical care programme, particularly in a field as specialised as neonatology. Their aim is not only to ensure the safety and well-being of newborn babies, but also to strengthen the confidence of parents and ensure open communication between medical staff and families.

Raising awareness to take action :
Awareness-raising is not simply the transmission of information. It is a process aimed at awakening people's attention and awareness to specific issues, in order to prompt them to take action. In the context of neonatology, this could mean raising parents' awareness of the importance of skin-to-skin contact, the signs of infection in a premature baby, or the impact of environmental stimuli on a baby's development.

Information sessions, leaflets, educational videos or interactive workshops can be organised to raise awareness of best practice in neonatology among parents and staff.

Educating for understanding :
Education, on the other hand, is more far-reaching. It aims to equip individuals with the knowledge and skills they need to understand and manage complex situations. Parents of premature babies can feel overwhelmed and anxious. Educating them about their child's specific needs, available treatments and long-term prospects can help them feel more in control and actively involved in their child's care.

Implementation :

Training sessions: Organise regular information sessions for parents on key subjects such as feeding premature babies, vital signs to look out for and stimulating development.

Teaching materials: Provide parents with brochures, books and reliable online resources so that they can learn at their own pace.

Interactive workshops: Organise workshops where parents can learn by doing, such as baby massage techniques or breastfeeding methods.

Feedback: Invite parents who have already been through the neonatal experience to share their stories, to offer hope and perspective to new families.

Ongoing evaluation: Make sure the information is understood and applied by carrying out regular evaluations and providing space for questions.

Raising awareness and educating are not limited to parents. Medical staff must also be continually trained and updated on the latest advances in neonatology. This culture of constant learning ensures that every member of the team is equipped to provide the best possible care, while also being a valuable guide to the families they serve.

Chapter 30:
DENTAL CARE IN NEONATOLOGY

The importance
of oral health from birth

Oral health is an essential part of overall health, and it starts at birth. Although newborn babies don't yet have teeth, the way we look after their mouths can have a lasting impact on their dental health throughout their lives. Here's why oral health is so important right from the start, and how it translates into habits that promote a lifetime of healthy smiles.

The foundations of oral health from birth :
   Preventing baby bottle tooth decay: Although they are temporary, baby teeth play a crucial role in oral health. They help with chewing, pronunciation and conserving space for future permanent teeth. Baby bottle tooth decay can occur when sugary liquids, such as milk, infant formula or juice, remain in prolonged contact with milk teeth. By starting with good oral hygiene from birth, you can prevent these cavities from appearing.
   Preparing for permanent teeth: Even before milk teeth begin to emerge, permanent teeth are already forming beneath the surface. A healthy mouth from an early age provides a favourable environment for these teeth to develop properly.
   Healthy eating habits: Introducing oral-healthy foods from the start, such as fibre-rich vegetables and calcium-rich dairy products, can help establish eating habits that promote healthy teeth.

How to promote oral health from birth:

Gentle cleaning: Even before the first tooth appears, it's a good idea to gently clean your baby's gums with moist gauze or a soft cloth after meals to eliminate bacteria.

First visit to the dentist: It is generally recommended that children see their dentist before their first birthday. This first visit establishes a basis for regular dental care throughout life.

Fluoride: Fluoride strengthens tooth enamel and prevents cavities. Your dentist can advise you on the need for fluoride supplements, depending on your age and requirements.

Balanced diet: Avoiding sugary foods and drinks and focusing on a diet rich in nutrients contributes to optimal oral health.

Preventing harmful habits: It's essential to avoid or limit habits such as thumb-sucking or prolonged dummy use, which can affect jaw growth and tooth alignment.

Oral health from birth is about more than clean teeth. It's the foundation on which a lifetime of oral well-being is built. By instilling healthy habits from the start, we give our children the tools they need to take care of their smiles at every stage of their lives.

Prevention and education for parents

Prevention and education for parents are an essential pillar in ensuring the health and well-being of children from their earliest days. Understanding the challenges of prevention means recognising that each stage of a child's development offers unique opportunities to establish healthy habits, appropriate care and careful monitoring.

As soon as pregnancy is announced, future parents find themselves immersed in a new world, full of discoveries but also of responsibilities. Education begins here: how to ensure the mother's well-being during pregnancy, what are the signs of healthy foetal development, how to prepare for childbirth. But this education doesn't stop at birth; it's only just beginning.

The first few months of a baby's life are crucial. Parents learn to interpret their child's needs, to distinguish between a cry of hunger and one of pain. They discover the importance of sleep, nutrition and first aid. And this is where prevention comes into its own. By understanding their newborn's basic needs, parents can anticipate and avoid many common problems, from colic to diaper rash.

But beyond primary care, prevention also encompasses broader aspects. How do you create a safe environment for a child who is starting to crawl and then walk? What toys are suitable for each age group, and how can accidents in the home be avoided? Prevention also means raising parents' awareness of the importance of vaccinations, recognising the symptoms of a food allergy and learning first aid techniques.

Educating parents also means preparing them for their new role, helping them to understand the emotions that run through them, to manage fatigue, stress and sometimes the baby blues. It means giving them the tools they need to build a healthy relationship with their child, to understand the basics of child psychology, and to support their little one as he makes his first emotional discoveries.

Finally, prevention and education also mean creating a community. It means recognising that a child's education does not rest solely on the shoulders of his or her parents, but is part of a wider dynamic in which health professionals, extended family, friends and even society as a whole all play a role. Every intervention, every piece of advice, every moment of sharing helps to build the solid foundations on which a child can flourish.

So prevention and parent education are much more than just guidelines: they represent a collective commitment to the health, safety and happiness of the next generation.

Collaboration with paediatric dentists

Working closely with paediatric dentists is essential to ensuring that the health of newborns and young children is looked after as a whole. This collaboration is part of an interdisciplinary approach in which each specialist contributes his or her expertise to the child's overall well-being.

From the very first weeks of life, healthcare professionals have a key role to play in educating parents about their child's oral health. Long before the first tooth appears, it is important to make parents aware of healthy practices, such as avoiding sugary night feeds, which can be a factor in early infant caries. Paediatric dentists can provide valuable information on appropriate care, brushing and even the importance of a first visit to the dentist before the child's first birthday.

Collaboration does not stop at prevention. In the case of oral pathologies or malformations, joint treatment with a paediatric dentist is essential. For example, a tongue-tie (ankyloglossia) can cause breastfeeding problems in newborn babies. An exchange between the paediatrician, the lactation consultant and the paediatric dentist can lead to better care for the baby.

In addition, certain medical conditions can have implications for oral health. Children with congenital heart disease, for example, may require special attention before any invasive dental procedures because of the risk of infective endocarditis. Similarly, certain drugs administered to newborns can affect dental development, requiring early monitoring and intervention.

Paediatric dentists can also play a key role in the early detection of certain diseases. Abnormalities of the teeth or oral mucosa may be the first signs of systemic or genetic disorders. Fluid communication between the paediatric dentist and the neonatologist can facilitate early diagnosis and appropriate treatment.

The collaboration between neonatology professionals and paediatric dentists is a natural symbiosis that aims to ensure optimum health for the child from its very first days. By contributing their know-how and expertise, each specialist contributes to a complete and harmonious care pathway for the well-being of the child and the peace of mind of the parents.

Chapter 31:
THE CHALLENGES OF PAIN
AND SEDATION

Pain assessment and management in newborn babies

Assessing and managing pain in newborn babies is of paramount importance, as untreated pain can have long-term consequences for a child's development. Contrary to some long-held beliefs, newborn babies, including premature babies, do feel pain. Recognising and treating this pain appropriately is therefore essential to their well-being.

Assessment of pain in newborns :
Assessing pain in newborns is based mainly on behavioural and physiological observations. Several pain assessment scales have been developed specifically for newborns, such as the EDIN scale (Newborn Pain and Discomfort Scale) and the NIPS scale (Neonatal Infant Pain Scale). These scales take into account various indicators such as facial expressions (grimace, frown), crying, body movements, changes in heart rate or oxygen saturation.

Pain management :
    Non-pharmacological interventions :
        Skin-to-skin contact: Also known as the Kangaroo method, direct contact between the mother's (or father's) skin and that of the baby has been shown to reduce the perception of pain during painful procedures.
        Breast-feeding or administration of sugar solutions: Sugar (such as sucrose)

administered before a painful procedure may reduce the pain felt by the baby.

Soothing environment: Reducing light and sound stimuli and wrapping the baby in a secure environment can help reduce stress and pain.

Dummies: Sucking can be soothing for newborns.

Pharmacological interventions :

Analgesics: Medicines such as paracetamol or ibuprofen can be used, always on prescription and with particular attention to dosage.

Local anaesthetics: These can be used for specific procedures to numb a localised area.

Sedation: In some cases, mild sedation may be necessary, especially if the baby is to undergo a more invasive procedure.

The importance of training and education :
It is essential that all healthcare professionals working in neonatology are trained to recognise the signs of pain in newborn babies and to use the appropriate assessment scales. A multidisciplinary approach, involving doctors, nurses, pharmacists and other specialists, will ensure optimum management of newborn pain.

Recognising and appropriately managing pain in newborn babies is fundamental to their well-being and development. An approach combining non-pharmacological and pharmacological interventions, tailored to each situation, will ensure the baby's comfort and reduce the potential negative effects of untreated pain.

Judicious use of sedatives and analgesics

The use of sedatives and analgesics in neonatology is a sensitive issue that requires careful attention. These drugs have essential roles, particularly in ensuring the comfort of the newborn during painful or stressful procedures and in treating specific medical conditions. However, their use requires careful consideration of the benefits versus the risks, particularly in newborns who have a nervous system that is still developing and a physiology that is distinct from that of adults.

Benefits of sedatives and analgesics :

Pain and stress reduction: These medicines can reduce the pain experienced during procedures such as venipuncture, intubation or surgery.

Physiological stability: They can help stabilise parameters such as heart rate, breathing and blood pressure during stressful situations.

Facilitating care: In some cases, sedation may be necessary for medical interventions on agitated or unstable newborns.

Associated risks :

Side effects: Newborns may experience adverse reactions to medicines, such as respiratory depression, cardiac disturbances or effects on blood pressure.

Neurological toxicity: Some studies suggest that prolonged or repeated exposure to sedatives and analgesics may have consequences for the cerebral development of newborn babies.

Dependence and withdrawal syndrome: Neonates with prolonged exposure to certain drugs, such as opioids, may develop dependence and present withdrawal symptoms when treatment is stopped.

Recommendations for judicious use :

- **Accurate pain assessment:** Before any administration, it is essential to assess the newborn's pain or stress using validated assessment tools.

- **Choosing the right drug: The** most appropriate drug for the situation must be selected, taking into account the side-effect profile and potential interactions with other treatments.

- **Appropriate dosage:** The dosage must be precisely adjusted according to the weight and gestational age of the newborn, and it is crucial to regularly monitor the baby's response to treatment.

- **Close monitoring:** Neonates receiving sedatives or analgesics should be carefully monitored, with regular measurements of their physiological parameters and observation of their neurological state.

- **Minimising the duration of treatment:** It is advisable to limit the duration of exposure to sedatives and analgesics as much as possible and to regularly review the appropriateness of continuing them.

- **Education and communication:** Parents must be informed of the reasons for administering these drugs, their potential benefits and the associated risks.

Sedatives and analgesics have an indisputable place in neonatal medicine, but their use must be judicious, carefully considered and based on an ongoing assessment of the benefits and risks for each newborn.

Non-pharmacological techniques to relieve pain

In the neonatal context, pain can have long-term adverse effects on brain development and behaviour. Fortunately, a variety of non-pharmacological techniques have been developed to help alleviate pain in newborns. These methods offer the advantage of minimising the use of drugs and their potential side-effects, while providing effective pain relief.

Skin-to-skin contact (Kangaroo method): This technique, in which the newborn is placed on the mother's or father's bare chest, has shown positive effects in terms of stabilising the heart rate, improving oxygenation and reducing pain.

Breastfeeding or sugar solution: Breastfeeding during painful procedures or administering a sugar solution may reduce signs of pain in newborns.

Non-nutritive soother: Sucking has calming and analgesic effects on babies.

Wrapping or gentle restraint: Wrapping the baby in a blanket or sheet, allowing him to move his hands towards his face, can provide a sense of security and reduce the perception of pain.

Tactile stimulation: Gentle massage or therapeutic touch can reduce stress and pain.

Music therapy: Soft music or lullabies, often chosen by parents, can have a calming effect and reduce pain.

Calm environment: Reducing light and sound stimuli around children can reduce their stress levels and, consequently, their perception of pain.

Comfortable positioning: Placing the baby in a natural, comfortable position, using cushions or rolls, can help reduce discomfort.

Parental presence: Simply having a parent nearby, speaking softly or singing, can be soothing for the baby.

Soothing scents: Some studies have suggested that the smell of a mother, for example, can have calming properties for newborn babies.

Behavioural interventions: These may include distraction techniques, such as the use of pictures or visual toys, to take the baby's attention away from the pain.

It is essential to note that the effectiveness of these techniques can vary from one newborn to another. In addition, a combination of several methods can often be more effective than a single technique. Finally, it is crucial to constantly monitor the baby's reaction to ensure that the technique is well tolerated and effective. Training and education of carers and parents in these techniques is essential to ensure optimal management of pain in newborns.

Chapter 32:
THE ROLE OF MUSIC
AND ART IN NEONATOLOGY

Positive impact of music therapy and art therapy

Music therapy and art therapy are two forms of expressive therapy that harness the respective powers of music and the visual arts to promote healing, well-being and personal growth. Both therapies offer a variety of benefits to diverse populations, from infants to the elderly. They are particularly valuable in contexts where words alone may not be sufficient to express emotions or experiences. Here is a fluid exploration of the positive impacts of these two therapies:

At the heart of a room lit by soft daylight, the melodies of an instrument resonate, captivating the attention of all present. This is a common scene in music therapy, a discipline that explores the depth of the relationship between people and music. The vibrations and melodies of music have the power to stimulate our brains, soothe our souls and revitalise our spirits. Whether for patients with neurological disorders, children with special needs or elderly people struggling with loneliness, music therapy offers a lifeline, helping them to express repressed emotions, improve their cognitive skills and even strengthen their motor functions.

Meanwhile, in another space, the fresh smell of paint wafts through the air. Hands of all ages are at work, transforming white canvases into kaleidoscopes of colour and emotion. Art therapy offers a refuge where traumas, anxieties and dreams can be depicted, often revealing hidden perspectives and realities. For those who find it difficult to verbalise their feelings, art becomes their voice, a means of expressing what is too deep or painful to put into words. Art therapy can boost self-esteem, build resilience and offer a sense of achievement.

By combining music and art, these unconventional therapies often transcend the barriers of language and culture. They offer avenues for healing that traditional methods can sometimes overlook. In a world where pain and suffering are often internalised, music and art therapy remind us of the importance of expression, offering a glimmer of hope to those in search of inner peace and harmony.

Implementation in the units neonatology

The introduction of music and art therapy in neonatal units may seem unexpected, but these approaches offer remarkable benefits for both newborn babies and their parents. In an environment often marked by the beeping of machines, dimmed lights and an atmosphere of anxiety, gentle music and artistic creativity can bring a touch of normality and comfort. Here's how these therapies can be used in such a setting:

Music therapy :
> **Lullabies and gentle songs**: Parents are encouraged to sing to their baby. The sound of the parent's voice, particularly the mother's, can stabilise the infant's heart and breathing rhythms and strengthen the parent-child bond.
> **Soft instruments**: Instruments such as Tibetan bowls, bells or xylophones with soft tones can be

played near the incubator, providing a soothing melody that contrasts with the usual sounds of the unit.

Recorded music: carefully selected playlists of gentle tunes can be played at low volume for newborns, helping them to relax and fall asleep.

Art therapy :

Parental creations: Parents can be encouraged to create works of art for their baby, such as drawings or collages, which can be placed near the incubator. This not only allows them to feel involved in their child's care, but also to manage their own stress.

Photography: Artistic photography of newborns can be a wonderful way to celebrate every little victory in their growth journey. It gives parents a different, positive perspective on the situation.

Journaling: Encouraging parents to keep a diary of their feelings, hopes and worries can serve as an emotional outlet, helping to process the neonatal experience.

The most important thing when using these therapies in neonatology is to ensure the safety and well-being of the newborn. Music must never be too loud, and all interactions must be adapted to the individual needs of each child. Finally, the therapists working in these units must be trained specifically in neonatology, understanding the unique needs of these patients and their families.

Feedback and case studies

In neonatology, feedback and case studies are essential to highlight the challenges and successes encountered in the care of newborn babies, and to provide a solid basis for improving practice. Here's how these stories and studies can shed light on the neonatal landscape:

Feedback :

Parents: Testimonials from parents who have been through a neonatal experience offer valuable insights. They can talk about their anxieties, the way they were supported by the medical team, or the highlights of their stay.

Medical staff: Nurses, doctors and other healthcare professionals can share their own challenges and successes, as well as the lessons they have learned from particular situations. This feedback can influence future protocols and training.

Former patients: As adults, children can sometimes look back on their experiences as premature babies or neonatal patients, offering a unique and inspiring perspective.

Case studies :

Complication management : A detailed study of a case where a newborn presented with rare complications can be a learning tool for professionals. How was the situation identified? What interventions were implemented? What was the outcome?

Innovative interventions: Describing a case where a new technique or therapy has been used successfully can serve as a model for other neonatal units.

Ethical decisions: Cases where particularly difficult decisions have had to be made, whether ethical dilemmas or situations involving several medical specialities, can provide opportunities for learning about communication, collaboration and ethics.

Holistic and alternative care: Presenting cases where non-conventional approaches, such as music therapy or therapeutic touch, have been successfully integrated into a patient's care plan may encourage other units to explore these methods.

Feedback and case studies offer a concrete way of learning, evolving and constantly improving neonatal care. These stories and studies embody the reality of the field's challenges and triumphs, highlighting the complexity and beauty of neonatal medicine.

Chapter 33:
THE IMPORTANCE
OF CONTINUITY CARE

Ensuring a smooth transition between different levels of care

Ensuring a smooth transition between different levels of care is crucial, not only for the continuity and quality of care provided to patients, but also for reducing the anxiety of families and patients themselves. This transition is often at the crossroads of a multitude of challenges, ranging from coordination between different healthcare professionals to understanding and acceptance by patients and their families. Here are a few key elements to ensure that it goes smoothly.

1. Effective communication :
Communication is the cornerstone of any successful transition. Healthcare professionals at both levels of care (where the patient has come from and where they are going) need to communicate effectively to ensure that all relevant details are passed on.

2. Advance planning :
A successful transition cannot be improvised. It requires careful planning, taking into account the patient's medical, emotional and social needs.

3. Patient and family education :
Patients and their families need to be fully informed about what to expect during the transition. This includes information about the new care setting, what might be different and what they should do if something goes wrong.

4. Interprofessional coordination :
The transition between different levels of care often involves a variety of healthcare professionals - from doctors and nurses to social workers and therapists. Close coordination between these professionals is essential.

5. Post-transition follow-up :
Regular monitoring after the transition ensures that patients adapt well to their new care environment and enables any problems to be identified and resolved quickly.

6. Full documentation :
All relevant details of the patient's medical history, current treatments, needs and preferences must be carefully documented and communicated at the time of transition.

7. Taking emotional needs into account :
The transition between different levels of care can be a stressful time for patients and their families. Offering emotional support, whether through counsellors, support groups or other resources, is therefore crucial.

8. Continuing professional development :
Healthcare professionals must be regularly trained in best practice in care transition, to ensure that the process runs as smoothly and efficiently as possible.

A smooth transition between different levels of care requires a holistic approach, which takes into account patients' medical, emotional and social needs. With careful planning, effective communication and appropriate training, it is possible to ensure that patients receive the care they need, when they need it.

Collaboration between professionals for optimum continuity

Collaboration between professionals is at the heart of contemporary medical care. It is essential to guarantee optimum continuity of care, avoid duplication, reduce medical errors and ensure a better understanding of the patient's overall needs. Let's approach this collaboration in a fluid and inclusive way.

Imagine a carefully choreographed ballet. On stage, each dancer is essential to the harmony of the performance, bringing his or her own unique touch to create the whole picture. In medicine, this complex dance is orchestrated every day between different professionals. From GPs to nurses, pharmacists to physiotherapists, each professional brings his or her specific expertise to the bedside.

In this medical symphony, communication plays the role of conductor. Transparent and regular information sharing is crucial to ensure that everyone involved is on the same wavelength. This involves multidisciplinary consultation meetings, clear medical reports and high-performance technological tools, such as electronic medical records, which provide rapid and reliable access to patient information.

But beyond simple communication, true collaboration requires mutual trust and deep respect. Each professional must recognise the value of the others, understand their skills and expertise, and be prepared to learn from them. It's a dance of equals, where ego is put aside in favour of the patient's well-being.

What's more, this collaboration is not limited to the walls of the hospital or doctor's surgery. It extends into the community, sometimes involving social workers, teachers or family members. It recognises that a patient's well-being is influenced by many factors, from their socio-economic situation to their family environment.

Continuing education also plays a key role in this collaborative journey. Healthcare professionals not only need to stay up to date in their own field, but also understand the basics of the other disciplines with which they interact. Interdisciplinary workshops and joint seminars can help bridge this gap.

The patient is at the centre of this collaboration. They are not simply spectators, but key players in this dance. Healthcare professionals must strive to include patients in discussions, to understand their needs, concerns and wishes, and to consider them as full partners in their own care.

So when all these elements come together - communication, respect, ongoing training and the active participation of the patient - collaboration between professionals can truly flourish, guaranteeing optimal continuity of care and the best possible outcome for each patient.

Implications for training and practice

Interprofessional collaboration is not an innate skill. It has to be acquired and perfected. In neonatology, as in other medical disciplines, training and practice are crucial to facilitating this collaboration. When we consider the implications of this collaboration for training and practice, several key elements stand out.

1. Integration of interprofessional education :
It is essential that medical and educational institutions

integrate interprofessional education from the start of medical studies. This enables students in medicine, nursing, pharmacy, physiotherapy and other related specialities to learn side by side, understand each other's roles and develop communication and teamwork skills.

2. Simulations and case studies:

The use of simulations and case studies enables professionals to put themselves in situations and learn how to interact in real-life scenarios. This reinforces not only technical skills, but also interpersonal and communication skills.

3. Encouraging continuing education :

Medicine is evolving rapidly, as are collaborative approaches. Professionals therefore need to engage in ongoing training to keep up to date with best practice, new technologies and trends in collaboration.

4. Creating a culture of mutual respect:

Clinical practice should encourage a culture where all team members are valued and respected. This includes recognising each other's skills and contributions and creating an environment where everyone feels comfortable sharing their opinions and concerns.

5. Establishing effective communication systems :

A strong communication system is crucial to successful collaboration. This could include regular team meetings, the use of integrated electronic medical records, and clear protocols for sharing information.

6. Involvement of patients and families :

Patients and their families are essential members of the care team. Professionals must therefore be trained to communicate effectively with them, to understand their needs and concerns, and to include them in the decision-making process.

7. Evaluation and feedback :

Finally, as with any skill, interprofessional collaboration needs to be regularly evaluated. Team members should be encouraged to give and receive constructive feedback in order to continue to grow and improve.

Interprofessional collaboration is both an art and a science, requiring both formal training and thoughtful practice. By integrating these elements into medical training and practice, we can ensure that all team members work together smoothly and seamlessly to provide the best possible care.

Chapter 34:
CONTINUING EDUCATION
AND FUTURE PROSPECTS

The importance of updating skills

In a world where technology, science and society are evolving at a frenetic pace, updating skills has become an inescapable necessity for every professional. Whether in the medical field, IT, education or any other sector, yesterday's knowledge can quickly become obsolete today. Keeping up to date is therefore vital to ensuring relevance, efficiency and safety in professional practice.

Responding to the rapid evolution of technology and science: Technological and scientific advances are constant. What was considered up-to-date information or techniques a few years ago can now be replaced by new methods or technologies.

Ensuring safety: In the medical field, for example, using old methods or ignoring the latest discoveries could potentially endanger patients' lives. In industry, not knowing the latest safety standards can lead to accidents.

Increasing employability: In a competitive labour market, those who invest in updating their skills are more likely to be hired, to progress in their careers and to keep their jobs.

Adapting to a changing environment: Society is changing, as are the needs and expectations of customers and patients. To stay relevant and respond to changing needs, it's essential to keep learning and evolving.

Improving self-confidence: Mastering the latest skills and knowledge in your field gives you the confidence to tackle professional challenges.

Promoting innovation: By keeping abreast of current trends, we can also anticipate future changes and innovate, rather than simply following the trend.

Meeting regulatory requirements: In many fields, there are regulatory or professional requirements that require ongoing training.

Commitment to professionalism: Updating skills reflects a commitment to professionalism, demonstrating a determination to offer the best possible service or care.

Upgrading skills is not a luxury, it's a necessity. It takes time, effort and sometimes financial resources, but the benefits - both for the individual and for society as a whole - are inestimable. Not only does it ensure relevance and competence in a changing world, it also contributes to ongoing personal and professional growth.

Advances in neonatology : being at the cutting edge

In the vast medical world, neonatology - the care of newborn babies, particularly premature babies - has seen remarkable advances over the decades. Being at the cutting edge in neonatology means not only keeping up with these developments, but also anticipating and participating in the next wave of innovations. Here's a fluid overview of the evolution of this field and its importance in today's medical landscape.

The first neonatal intensive care units (NICUs) marked a revolution in the care of newborn babies, particularly premature babies. Previously, the chances of survival for a baby born prematurely were minimal. Today, thanks to technological, diagnostic and therapeutic advances, these little fighters not only have a chance of survival, but also a prospect of a quality life.

Neonatal respirators, for example, have undergone considerable improvements, allowing gentler ventilation and minimising lung damage. Nutrition, which plays a crucial role in the development of these babies, has become more personalised, taking into account the specific needs of each child. Advances in enteral and parenteral nutrition have enhanced growth and neurological development.

Pharmacology is no exception. Understanding the specific pharmacokinetics of newborns has led to more accurate dosing and safer administration of drugs, thereby reducing side effects.

Beyond technology and medicine, the family-centred approach has introduced a holistic dimension to neonatal care. Recognising the crucial role of parents and families, this approach encourages the active participation of parents in care, strengthening the parent-child bond from the very beginning.

But with all progress comes new challenges. Constant innovation requires ongoing training for medical staff, ensuring that the care they provide is at the cutting edge of science and technology. Professionals must also navigate the delicate waters of ethics, particularly when it comes to making decisions about life and death.

Research in neonatology is constantly evolving. Recent studies have explored the beneficial effects of complementary therapies, such as music therapy or therapeutic touch, on newborn babies in the NICU.

Genetics, too, offers exciting prospects for the early diagnosis and management of congenital anomalies.

Being at the cutting edge of progress in neonatology means having one foot firmly planted in current advances while keeping an eye on the horizon of future possibilities. It's a delicate dance between science, technology, ethics and humanity, and it demands passion, dedication and a constant willingness to learn and innovate.

Career opportunities and specialisations

Neonatology, a specialist branch of paediatrics, offers a fascinating range of career opportunities for those who are passionate about caring for newborn babies. Let's take a look at the various career opportunities and specialisations in this field.
The most obvious career in neonatology is that of neonatologist. These specialist doctors are dedicated to the care of newborn babies, particularly premature babies or those with complications at birth. To become a neonatologist, you need basic medical training followed by a specialisation in paediatrics and then a sub-specialisation in neonatology.

However, the world of neonatology is not limited to medicine. There are a multitude of professionals working in synergy to ensure the well-being of babies. Neonatal nurses, for example, play a crucial role in the day-to-day care and monitoring of newborn babies. They are often the first point of contact for families and offer essential support to parents at this delicate time.

Physiotherapists specialising in neonatal care are trained to work with newborns who require respiratory assistance or who have specific needs in terms of mobility and muscle development. They work closely with doctors to develop appropriate care plans.

In addition, given the delicate and often stressful nature of this field, psychologists and social workers also play an essential role. They support families through the emotional and social challenges, providing advice, resources and a space to process the complex emotions associated with the birth of a premature or sick child.

Other specialities that interact closely with neonatology include medical genetics, paediatric cardiology, paediatric surgery and paediatric neurology. Each specialist brings unique expertise to bear on a range of complications or conditions.

Outside the clinical context, there are opportunities for researchers with a passion for neonatology. Universities, research institutes and even some large hospital units offer positions for those wishing to push back the frontiers of knowledge in this field.

Finally, for those with a penchant for teaching, there is a demand for neonatal trainers, whether in medical schools, nursing training programmes or professional development workshops.

Neonatology is a rich and multi-dimensional field that offers a multitude of careers for those seeking to make a difference in the crucial first moments of human life. Every role, whether directly medical or supportive, contributes to the enormous task of ensuring the best possible start in life for these little ones.

Conclusion

The neonatal vocation :
more than a job, a passion

Neonatology, a sphere dedicated to the very first moments of life, resonates far beyond the boundaries of a simple medical profession. For those who choose it, it embodies a profound vocation, a passion that goes far beyond simple clinical practice. Let's sail together through this wonderful quest for meaning and dedication.

When you enter a neonatal care unit, the first thing you feel is that special atmosphere, charged with contrasting emotions. There's the silent joy that accompanies every heartbeat you hear, every little hand that clasps a finger, every smile as a mother holds her child for the first time. But there is also the palpable tension, the weight of responsibility that accompanies every decision, every intervention. In this ballet, the neonatal staff move with unfailing grace and determination.

This vocation is often born from a spark, sometimes from personal experience, or simply from a fascination for the miracles of new life. It's the desire to stand at the frontier of life, where it all begins, to be the guardian of these new souls, the guide for these families in the midst of upheaval. Every professional in neonatology, whether doctor, nurse, psychologist or other, pursues this quest with boundless dedication.

But what fuels this passion? Is it seeing these tiny creatures, so fragile yet so resilient, struggle every day? Is it the immeasurable love in their parents' eyes, that glimmer of hope and gratitude? Or is it simply the beauty inherent in this beginning of life, the innocence and purity that remind us all of the priceless value of each moment?

Neonatology is not simply a matter of technical skills and medical knowledge, although these are crucial. Above all, it is a matter of the heart. It requires sensitivity, empathy and the inner strength to face heartbreaking situations, but also to celebrate every little victory, every step forward.

And it is in this fusion of science and soul, skill and compassion, that the true essence of the neonatal vocation lies. It's not just a profession, it's a deep commitment to life, an oath to accompany, protect and cherish these precious beginnings. For those who choose this path, neonatology becomes more than a profession: it becomes an integral part of their being, a constant echo of their love for life and for humanity.

Encouraging the next generation: the future of neonatology

In the subdued light of a neonatal unit, where every second counts and every gesture can be life-saving, the future of these little ones takes shape. But at the same time, another future is also taking shape: that of neonatology itself. Encouraging the next generation of carers to immerse themselves in this speciality, to embrace its challenges and carry its banner, is essential to ensure that newborn care continues to progress.

Neonatology, with its rapid technological advances and scientific discoveries, is constantly evolving. This dynamic requires a new generation of professionals who are passionate, dedicated and, above all, trained in the latest techniques and knowledge. These young minds, with their freshness and curiosity, are the key to pushing back the frontiers of what we know and can do for newborn babies.

But how can we inspire and motivate these future pioneers of neonatology?

Telling the stories. Nothing is more powerful than sharing real stories, moments of triumph and tragedy, to show the profound impact of this profession. Every smile of a child who has survived against all the odds, every tear shed with a family in difficult times, is a testament to the importance of this profession.

Providing learning opportunities. Neonatal placements, practical workshops and research seminars allow students and young professionals to immerse themselves in the world of neonatology, learn from the best and discover their own passion.

Support and mentoring. Solid support from experienced professionals can make all the difference to a young professional's career. A mentor can not only provide knowledge, but also inspire, encourage and guide.

Highlighting innovation. The new generation was born in the digital age and is familiar with technology and innovation. By showing how neonatology is evolving thanks to technological advances, we can capture their interest and encourage them to be the innovators of tomorrow.

Encouraging the new generation means believing in the future. It's about recognising that, just like those babies who start life with so much potential, neonatology itself is at a point of growth, ready to be shaped by fresh, determined hands. The future of neonatology is bright, full of hope and promise, provided we pass the torch with passion and dedication.

The future of neonatology

The future of neonatology, a medical speciality already at the cutting edge of technology and innovation, promises to be a fascinating convergence of technological advances, new therapeutic approaches and an even deeper understanding of the needs of newborn babies.

1. Advanced technologies: The future will see a growing adoption of technologies such as artificial intelligence and robotics to aid early diagnosis and treatment of neonatal conditions. Connected monitors could offer real-time surveillance, detecting the early signs of a problem long before it becomes visible.

2. Genomics and personalised therapies: As genetic sequencing becomes more accessible, it will be possible to detect genetic anomalies and offer personalised treatments from the very first days of life.

3. Less invasive techniques: New, less invasive and more precise intervention methods will be developed, reducing stress and risks for the newborn while increasing the chances of success.

4. Biotechnology: 3D printing could make it possible to create tailor-made organs or tissues to replace defective ones in newborn babies.

5. Optimal environment: Increased research into the importance of the newborn's environment (light, sound, touch) will lead to neonatal units that are even more patient-centred, offering an atmosphere as close as possible to that of the womb.

6. Greater role for parents: A better understanding of the importance of the parent-child bond in the healing process will lead to parents becoming even more involved in care, by training and supporting them at every stage.

7. Holistic approaches: Recognition of the benefits of non-conventional methods, such as music therapy or therapeutic touch, could become an integral part of standard treatment in neonatology.

8. Interdisciplinary collaboration: The future will see even closer collaboration between neonatologists, nurses, psychologists, therapists and other specialists, ensuring comprehensive care for the newborn.

9. Tele-neonatology: With the expansion of telemedicine, specialists will be able to offer advice and consultations at a distance, ensuring that newborns, wherever they are, have access to the best possible care.

The future of neonatology is emerging as an era of integrated care, where technology, science and humanity converge to give newborn babies the best possible start in life. Although faced with challenges, with the passion and dedication of those working in this field, the future of neonatal care looks bright.

Technological advances on the horizon

The last decade has seen an exponential proliferation of innovative technologies in a variety of fields, and this trend looks set to intensify in the future. Whether in health, energy, transport or communications, technological advances are shaping our future in ways we could never have imagined before. Here are some of the most promising technological advances on the horizon:

1. Artificial Intelligence (AI) and Machine Learning: Although these technologies are not new, they are becoming increasingly integrated into a variety of sectors. AI and machine learning can now diagnose diseases, manage complex energy systems and even compose music.

2. Biotechnology: CRISPR and other gene-editing techniques promise to revolutionise medicine, offering the possibility of curing genetic diseases and personalising medical treatments.

3. Augmented reality (AR) and virtual reality (VR): Beyond gaming, these technologies have enormous potential in vocational training, education, design and even medicine.

4. Clean energy: Research into batteries, nuclear fusion and other renewable energy sources suggests a future in which our dependence on fossil fuels could diminish.

5. Autonomous vehicles: From cars to delivery drones, autonomous vehicle technology could transform our transport systems and reduce road accidents.

6. Internet of Things (IoT): Connecting almost every device to the Internet can lead to smart cities, more efficient homes and a better understanding of our environment.

7. Neurotechnology: From brain-machine interfaces to the mapping of the human brain, advances in this field could transform the treatment of neurological diseases and perhaps even improve cognitive abilities.

8. 3D printing: Beyond the rapid manufacture of prototypes, 3D printing has the potential to revolutionise manufacturing, medicine (think printed organs) and even house building.

9. Nanotechnology: The use of particles on an incredibly small scale could have huge implications for medicine, energy and manufacturing.

10. 5G and beyond: As the roll-out of 5G gets underway, this technology promises ultra-fast download speeds, reduced latency and the ability to connect even more devices to the internet.

The technological horizon is vast and full of promise. Of course, with every advance comes its own set of challenges, whether ethical, economic or social. Nevertheless, as technology advances, it offers unprecedented opportunities to improve lives, solve age-old problems and open up new avenues for the future of humanity.

Current research
and its implications for practice

Research plays a fundamental role in the evolution of all fields, including neonatology. Breakthroughs in research determine best practice, provide invaluable insights into the care of newborns and influence the future direction of healthcare. Here's a look at how current research is influencing neonatal practice:

1. Feeding methods: Research has highlighted the extraordinary benefits of breast milk for preterm infants, particularly in the prevention of necrotising bowel disease. This awareness has encouraged many neonatal units to adopt proactive policies to support breastfeeding.

2. Neonatal microbiome: Studies have shown that the first bacteria to colonise a newborn baby's gut can have a lasting impact on its health. As a result, there is now growing interest in protecting and promoting a healthy microbiome in the newborn, particularly through the prudent use of antibiotics.

3. Impact of the environment : Research has shown the importance of a calm environment, with subdued light and minimal noise, for the development of the premature baby. This has led to changes in the design of neonatal care units.

4. Non-Pharmacological Approaches: Studies have highlighted the effectiveness of techniques such as therapeutic touch, music therapy and skin-to-skin contact (also known as the Kangaroo Method) in managing pain, comforting newborns and improving parent-child attachment.

5. Neuroprotection: Recent research focuses on the impact of care and interventions on the developing brain, leading to changes in the way care is delivered to minimise the risk of brain damage.

6. Minimally invasive procedures: Technological advances and research have led to minimally invasive procedures for surgical interventions, reducing the associated risks and speeding up recovery.

7. Ethics and Palliative Care: Research into ethics and families' experiences has shaped the way healthcare professionals approach difficult decisions, highlighting the importance of open communication, compassion and support when making decisions about end of life care.

Finally, it is crucial to recognise that, although research can guide practice, there is often a gap between the two. Integrating research findings into clinical practice requires ongoing education, awareness and a willingness to adapt care based on new knowledge. Research is a constant journey, and its impact on neonatology is constantly evolving, leading to better insights and better care for the most vulnerable among us.

Vision of the future: where could neonatology take us in the coming decades?

With the dawn of new scientific discoveries and technological innovations, neonatology holds out the promise of a future in which every newborn baby will have the chance of a healthy life, even in the face of adverse circumstances. But what directions might neonatology take in the decades ahead?

As our understanding of DNA and the human genome deepens, a new era of personalised medicine is emerging, offering undreamt-of possibilities. Imagine a world where, from the very first moments of life, every child benefits from genetic mapping to identify not only potential diseases, but also the best way to treat or even prevent them.

At the same time, biotechnology, with the advent of regenerative therapies, could open doors once considered impenetrable. Damaged tissues could be repaired, or even replaced, using laboratory-grown organs, giving premature babies a chance to correct malformations or dysfunctions before they even occur.

The integration of technology into neonatology will not stop there. With the rise of robotics and artificial intelligence, we can envisage neonatal units where robot assistants would take part in the care of newborns, monitoring vital signs in real time, anticipating needs and even detecting the first signs of infection or other complications.

The human dimension, however, will remain at the heart of this speciality. Technological advances will need to be harmonised with a holistic approach to care. Tomorrow's neonatal units will probably be designed to encourage even greater interaction between newborn babies, their families and the medical team. These environments, designed to ensure the well-being and emotional balance of all concerned, will contribute to faster and more serene recovery.

The neonatology of tomorrow, with its wealth of scientific advances and heightened human sensitivity, promises us a future where every newborn, whatever their initial challenges, will have the chance to blossom fully in the world that awaits them.

www.ingramcontent.com/pod-product-compliance
Lightning Source LLC
Chambersburg PA
CBHW072153290526
45794CB00004B/1505